PLANETARY HEALTH AND SOCIAL SECURITY

Offering an in-depth exploration of the security challenges posed by COVID-19, Gunaratna, Aslam, and their contributors present a comprehensive collection of thematic and country-specific analyses on post-pandemic planetary health strategies.

This book critically evaluates the global challenges and responses to COVID-19, examining its impact across key sectors such as security, defense, trade, health, economy, and religion. Through empirical evidence and diverse case studies, it analyzes the strengths and shortcomings of international efforts and offers thoughtful approaches and solutions to fostering a balanced and resilient planet for future generations.

Essential for students and scholars of planetary health, international relations, humanitarian affairs, strategic and defense management, policy studies, and global health, this book also serves as a valuable resource for policymakers, government ministries, and agencies seeking insights into effective global practices.

Mohd Mizan Aslam is Professor in Security & Strategic Studies at the National Defence University of Malaysia (NDUM) and Senior Fellow at the Global Peace Institute (GPI), London, United Kingdom.

Rohan Gunaratna is Professor of Security Studies at the S. Rajaratnam School of International Studies, Nanyang Technology University, and Founder of International Centre for Political Violence and Terrorism Research, Singapore.

"This book is essential reading for policymakers, students, and anyone invested in the future of our planet. It offers both a compelling narrative and practical solutions, demonstrating that the health of our planet and the security of our communities are inextricably linked. A must-read for those committed to creating a just, healthy, and sustainable world for all."

Dr. Fabian Sandor, *Deputy Regional Advisor for Europe and Africa, Irregular Warfare Centre, Washington DC*

"*Planetary Health and Social Security* presents a transformative analysis of the complex interdependencies between ecological systems and human well-being. By integrating perspectives from environmental science, public health, and social justice, the book critically examines pressing global challenges, including climate change, biodiversity loss, and social inequality, with particular attention to their disproportionate impacts on vulnerable populations.

"The authors propose an integrative framework for policymaking that emphasizes the dual imperatives of sustainability and equity. By addressing these interwoven issues holistically, the book seeks to advance innovative strategies and actionable solutions that promote long-term planetary health and social resilience.

"This scholarly work invites readers to reimagine humanity's relationship with the environment critically. It underscores the importance of collective, evidence-based efforts to secure a sustainable and equitable future for all."

Dr. Ilyas Mohamed-Derby, *University, UK*

"Through thorough research and compelling case studies, this book illuminates the urgent need for integrated policies that promote environmental sustainability and social justice simultaneously. It encourages readers to rethink traditional paradigms and embrace innovative solutions to the crises we face. This work serves as both a wake-up call and a guide, inspiring all stakeholders—from community activists to government leaders—to take action. The future of humanity depends on our ability to secure a healthy planet alongside our social structures, making this book an invaluable resource for anyone passionate about planetary preservation and social equity.

"COVID-19 was a wake-up call for every individual on the globe. Tackling the multi-faced and long-established problems observed and experienced globally is not easy. However, having a sustainable initiative, from the individual and communal to the regional and global, is undoubtedly crucial and will be crucial for the future of human and natural ecosystems."

Dr. Mehmet Özay, *ISTAC, IIUM Malaysia*

PLANETARY HEALTH AND SOCIAL SECURITY

Securing Our Common Future

*Edited by Mohd Mizan Aslam
and Rohan Gunaratna*

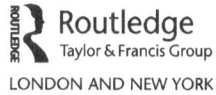
Routledge
Taylor & Francis Group

LONDON AND NEW YORK

Designed cover image: Getty Images

First published 2025
by Routledge
4 Park Square, Milton Park, Abingdon, Oxon OX14 4RN

and by Routledge
605 Third Avenue, New York, NY 10158

Routledge is an imprint of the Taylor & Francis Group, an informa business

British Library Cataloguing-in-Publication Data
A catalogue record for this book is available from the British Library

Library of Congress Cataloging-in-Publication Data
Names: Aslam, Mohd Mizan, editor. | Gunaratna, Rohan, 1961- editor.
Title: Planetary health and social security : securing our common future / edited by Mohd Mizan Aslam and Rohan Gunaratna.
Description: Abingdon, Oxon ; New York, NY : Routledge, [2025] | Includes bibliographical references and index. |
Identifiers: LCCN 2024062083 (print) | LCCN 2024062084 (ebook) |
ISBN 9781032941288 (hardback) | ISBN 9781032941271 (paperback) |
ISBN 9781003569084 (ebook)
Subjects: LCSH: Public health--International cooperation--Case studies. |
Public health--Safety measures--Case studies. | Human security--International cooperation--Case studies. | COVID-19 Pandemic, 2020-2023--Case studies.
Classification: LCC RA441 .P54 2025 (print) | LCC RA441 (ebook) |
DDC 362.1--dc23/eng/20250226
LC record available at https://lccn.loc.gov/2024062083
LC ebook record available at https://lccn.loc.gov/2024062084

ISBN: 978-1-032-94128-8 (hbk)
ISBN: 978-1-032-94127-1 (pbk)
ISBN: 978-1-003-56908-4 (ebk)

DOI: 10.4324/9781003569084

Typeset in Times New Roman
by KnowledgeWorks Global Ltd.

CONTENTS

ACKNOWLEDGMENTS

Mizan and Rohan would like to thank the contributing authors for participating in an unprecedented project. We are indebted for the valuable suggestions by the reviewers. In Singapore, we would like to express our gratitude by thanking our research assistants, Clifford Gere and Glenda Tan of the S. Rajaratnam School of International Studies and Rochelle Teo of the Department of Psychology, the Nanyang Technology University (NTU), Singapore. Our special thanks go to Vanessa Lim Panes, Vlad Antonio, Sievalee Wijayawardhana, and Tristan Muralitharan for their research assistance.

We would also like to thank Kasiviswanathan Shanmugam, Minister of Home Affairs of Singapore; Tito Karnavian, Minister of Home Affairs of Indonesia; and Dato' Seri Zambry Kadir, the Higher Education Minister of Malaysia for their vision. Many in governments both past and present, especially the visionary leadership Mr. Benny Lim, led to creating a research culture in security studies. Similarly, in Malaysia, our deepest appreciation goes to Deputy Inspector General of Malaysia, Datuk Ayob Khan Mydin Pitchay, and Lieutenant General (R) Datuk Hasagaya Abdullah, former Vice Chancellor of National Defence University of Malaysia for fostering cooperation between the government, community organizations, and academia.

We thank the staff of the International Centre for Political Violence and Terrorism Research (ICPVTR) at NTU, Singapore; the National Defence University of Malaysia (UPNM); and the Prime Minister's Office (PMO) for their steadfast assistance supporting research on national and international security threats and response during the pandemic.

FOREWORD

The COVID-19 pandemic matters to the whole world; while we can't predict exactly when or where the next outbreak will begin, we know one is coming in just a matter of time. Unprecedented tragedies in the modern world shocked every single country. It thereby appears that in managing such a threat, timely response is the key to success. It is essential to see defense as a premier frontliner, maintain mission readiness, ensure public safety, and support government-wide efforts in a wide range of areas by prompt and precise response to the threat of COVID-19. How we stop outbreaks from becoming widespread pandemics that threaten us all will be an indicator that ensures the sustainability of Malaysian citizens regardless of place and space.

COVID-19 takes hold in the world's most vulnerable areas, especially defense, education, health, food, religion, trade, and business activities. Countries with very little resources to stop the spread of infection before it reaches their shores will be left in bad situations. When a virus can travel from a secluded corner to major cities on all continents in less than two days, the threat to our national defense is greater than ever. Many challenges exist worldwide that increase the risk of pandemic and rapid spread, including the following:

- Acts of terrorism
- Digital acceleration
- Ability to travel
- Massive online trade and business
- Acts of bioterrorism
- Weaknesses of public health infrastructures
- Religious congregations and many more

The world must come forward together, taking steps to better detect, plan, and respond to COVID-19. Every single country has to develop a pre- and post-COVID-19 response system. This response will hold best practice that will allow better support in country's defense. A system of planning and responsiveness, including the immediate need to analyze the current COVID-19 outbreak and the impact on every single aspect of the country, also has to be developed.

With that, I congratulate Dr. Mizan and Dr. Rohan on getting your timely book published! Precious few have had the nerve to write on the COVID-19 threat and response. You have written an excellent book that should raise lots of eyebrows. Of course, many of your chapters were done by accomplished researchers and practitioners in the matter. Nevertheless, both of you must have done a wheelbarrow-full of research on pandemic threat and response across disciplines. I admire your academic work. I guess this means we will be seeing more of you in the print media from now on. I say congratulations to both of you!

Mr. Adly Zahari
Deputy Minister of Defence
Government of Malaysia

CONTRIBUTORS

Mohd Mizan Aslam holds a position as Professor in Security & Strategic Studies at the National Defence University of Malaysia (NDUM). Mizan is also a Senior Fellow at the Global Peace Institute (GPI), London, United Kingdom. Mizan holds a position at the National Panel for Deradicalization, a special task-force unit for rehabilitation for terrorist inmates. Mizan also works with the Prime Minister's Office & Ministry of Home Affairs of Malaysia in the field of research and developing modules and programs on deradicalization programs (PCVE). Mizan was a former professor in Counter Terrorism Studies at the Naif Arab University for Security Sciences (NAUSS), Riyadh Saudi Arabia, where he established the Centre for Terrorism & Extremism Studies (CTES). He holds the position of Chairman of Perdana Global Peace Foundation (PGPF). Mizan also works with the Middle Eastern Institute (MEI), Washington USA, as Country Expert in analyzing terrorism and extremism issues in SEA & MENA. He was a visiting scholar at University of Hawaii at Manoa, USA, and Ibnu Haldun Universitasi, Istanbul.

Efri Syamsul Bahri is a lecturer at the SEBI School of Islamic Economics, Indonesia. He is also a Master Trainer and Competency Assessor. He is also an editor and reviewer of scientific journals. He has authored scientific articles in human resource management, Zakat, and Waqf. He obtained a PhD in Business Administration from Asia e University, Selangor Malaysia. He received his Master's in Administration and Public Policy from Muhammadiyah University, Jakarta. He obtained a Bachelor's degree in accounting from Andalas University. He is also active in various organizations, including the Islamic Association of University Students (HMI) and the Indonesian Mosque Youth and Youth Communication Agency (BKPRMI). He has also written several books, including *Sustainable Community Empowerment*, *Concepts and Applications of Community Empowerment*, and

SROI: Social Return on Investment, a method of measuring the economic, environmental and social benefits (impact) of programs or projects.

Liu Chunlin is the founder of K&C Protective Technologies (KCPT), Singapore, since 2004. He has a doctorate in Management Science and Engineering (Tsinghua University), and another doctorate in Structural Engineering (Tongji University), as well as an MBA (National University of Singapore). Being a high achiever and having won many international competitions in technology innovations from Europe and the US over the past 35 years, Dr. Liu has also published several papers, reports, and books focused on blast and security engineering and construction technology. Following his interest in research and development, Dr. Liu owns several patents related to protective technologies, including risk assessment methodology, anti-crash system, enhanced protective films system, structural hardening, and cost modeling.

Nur Efendi, since 2012 has been CEO of Rumah Zakat, one of the largest philanthropic institutions in Indonesia. This man, born in Kudus on March 6 1981, completed his Bachelor's degree at UIN Walisongo Semarang and a Master's in Sharia Economics at UNISBA Bandung. He has achieved various achievements and recognition with Rumah Zakat, including bringing this institution to become The Biggest LAZ since 2014. In his hands, Rumah Zakat's performance has also made achievements at the world level by being recognized as an institution with special consultative status from the United Nations. In 2019 Nur Efendi was named Best CEO by *SWA* magazine and TOP Leader by *It Work* magazine, included in the ranks of top leaders of other large companies and people of the year 2021 by MetroTV. In the world of the Zakat movement, Nur Efendi was once the general chairman of the Zakat Forum (FOZ), an association of Zakat institutions in Indonesia. Nur Efendi's current position is on the Board of Trustees of Rumah Zakat, Chair of Syarikat Amil Indonesia, and Manager of the Association of Indonesian Islamic Economic Experts (IAEI). All this is to do good and be useful for others.

Rohan Gunaratna is Professor of Security Studies at the S. Rajaratnam School of International Studies, Nanyang Technology University, and Founder of International Centre for Political Violence and Terrorism Research, Singapore. He received his master's from the University of Notre Dame in the US, where he was a Hesburgh Scholar, and his doctorate from the University of St Andrews in the UK, where he was a British Chevening Scholar. A former Senior Fellow at the Combating Terrorism Centre at the United States Military Academy at West Point and the Fletcher School of Law and Diplomacy, Gunaratna was Visiting Fellow at the Washington Institute for Near East Policy. The author of *Inside al Qaeda: Global Network of Terror* (University of Columbia Press), Gunaratna edited the Insurgency and Terrorism Series of the Imperial College Press, London. A trainer for national security agencies, law enforcement authorities, and military counter-terrorism units, he interviewed terrorists and insurgents in Afghanistan, Pakistan, Iraq, Yemen, Libya, Saudi Arabia and other conflict zones. For advancing international security cooperation, Gunaratna received the Major General Ralph H. Van Deman Award.

John Harrison is an internationally recognized expert in terrorism, aviation security, and political violence. He is an Associate Professor at Rabdan Academy, where he served as senior faculty at the new Zayed Military University and assisted in developing Rabdan Academy's Bachelor's of Science in Homeland Security and the MS in Intelligence. Prior to Rabdan he was a senior analyst for CyberPoint International LLC. He was a professor for the National Defense University Program for the US Special Operations community at Fort Bragg. Previously he was the Head of Terrorism Research at the International Center for Political Violence and Terrorism Research in Singapore and served as the Coordinator of Transportation Security at the University's Center for Excellence in National Security. Dr. Harrison serves as an Associate Editor of the international *Journal of Transportation Security*. He has multiple publications, including his book, *International Aviation and Terrorism*, which was published in March 2009. He has been on the Editorial Board for the Institute of National Security Studies *Sri Lanka's Defense Review* and the International Advisory Board of the Global Peace Institute; as well as the Nordic Counter Terrorism Group, and the Southeast Asia Chapter of the International Association for Counterterrorism and Security Professionals. In 2008 Dr. Harrison was embedded with a US Military Transition Team in Tikrit, Iraq. Dr. Harrison earned a PhD in International Relations and an MLitt in International Security Studies from St Andrews University in Scotland. He has an MA in Political Science from the American University in Washington, DC and a BA in Political Science from Wheeling Jesuit University.

Kyounggun Kim has very strong experience in both the cybersecurity industry and academia for 20 years. He is currently an Assistant Professor, Department of Forensic Sciences, Naif Arab University for Security Sciences (NAUSS). He is a founding member of the Center of Excellence in Cybercrime and Digital Forensics (CoECDF) and head of the network forensics department. He teaches cybersecurity and cybercrime to higher diploma students at NAUSS. Before he joined the NAUSS, he lectured in offensive cyber capabilities to graduate and undergraduate students at Korea University from September 2016 to August 2020. He received the Excellent Teaching Award in Korea University (2018, 2019, and 2020). He is a representative security consulting mentor at the Best of the Best (BoB) program sponsored by the Korean government. He has been invited by the United Nations Office on Drugs and Crime (UNODC) as a lecturer for Western/Asian professors to promote the Education for Justice (E4J) initiative. He is a member of UNODC Education for Justice initiative network. He is reviewer for the Elsevier Computers and Security, IEEE Communications and Survey, IEEE Access, and ETRI journal. He has conducted penetration testing for over 130 clients for various industries such as financial, energy, and consumers when he worked for Deloitte, PwC, and boutique consulting firms for more than 15 years. He won a sixth-place prize in DefCon CTF 2007 and got a first prize at 1st Hacking Defense Contest hosted by Korea Information Security Agency. He has an extraordinary ability to lead students' enthusiasm to the best and achieve the best.

Pamungkas Hendra Kusuma is a dedicated humanitarian activist who began his career in the social world as a doctor at the free clinic of Rumah Zakat, right after graduating from the Faculty of Medicine at Universitas Padjadjaran in Bandung, Indonesia in 2003. His unwavering commitment to dedicating his life to social humanitarian work has led him to become the Director of the National Zakat Institution, where he is trusted as one of the leaders of the National Zakat Forum. Driven by concern for the conditions of communities in various remote areas of Indonesia, he has established several humanitarian institutions such as Insan Bumi Mandiri and Sahabat Pedalaman, as well as LAZ Sakinah Berkah. Dozens of Zakat and Humanitarian Social Institutions across Indonesia have recognized him as a consultant in facing rapid changes in the digital era. He is also the founder of the Koperasi Paguyuban Sakinah Berkah, which since 2017 has helped more than 3,000 families escape the clutches of loan sharks.

Muhd Nabhan Mizan is currently in his penultimate year at University College London. As a scholar of Politics and International Relations, his main focus of study is religion and politics, and political violence in Southeast Asia. Throughout Nabhan's years in college, he has actively engaged in student activism both in his hometown, in Malaysia, and the UK. His most recent experience was as the Head of Career and Talent Development with the National Council of Malaysians. Throughout his service, Nabhan has engaged with multiple organizations aiming to bridge students with the professional sector. His future endeavors are to develop and disseminate intellectual political knowledge for the masses.

Immanuel Azaad Moonesar is Professor of Health Policy and Systems Research at Mohammed Bin Rashid School of Government, Dubai, UAE. Prof. Moonesar hails from the Caribbean islands of Trinidad and Tobago and France, and he also serves as Managing Director at "I AM Consulting" (Trinidad & Tobago), and President (Chapter Chair) and Executive Board member of the Academy of International Business—Middle East North Africa (AIB-MENA). He is also a registered dietitian. Throughout his career, he has worked in quality assurance and management, nutrition and dietetics, health and safety, teaching, and institutional research. His research interests are well-being, mental health, IB policy, public policy, healthcare management and leadership, maternal and child health, health policy and innovation, nutrition, AI, and quality management. He also has more than 255+ publications in peer-reviewed journal articles, has presented papers at peer-reviewed international conferences, and has co-authored books, and book chapters. His research grants and fundraising attainment amount to over 4,000,000 USD.

Lihini Ratwatte is a development practitioner based in Sri Lanka. She has worked with government, private sector, non-governmental and international organizations, as well as with think tanks, research institutions, and development partners across Sri Lanka and the South Asian region. Ms. Ratwatte's professional expertise ranges from research, policy analysis, and advocacy to practical applications of gender, development, and governance across national, sub-national and grassroots levels in Sri Lanka. Ms. Ratwatte holds a Bachelor of Arts in International Studies, Communications and Gender Studies from Monash University (2014), and a Master of Arts in Global Diplomacy from SOAS – University of London (2017). Drawing from her academic and work experience, Ms. Ratwatte's research and academic discourse focuses on the nexus of gender, development, peacebuilding and security in the Asia-Pacific region.

Any Rufaedah is a senior lecturer at the Department of Psychology, Universitas Nahdlatul Ulama Jakarta and senior analyst at Division for Applied Social Psychology Research (DASPR). She is interested in the study of conflict, radicalism, terrorism, and women. Between 2015 and 2018, before receiving her research fellowship in the United States, she conducted intervention research with wives of terror convicts in various cities in Indonesia. She is currently completing a course in Strategic Studies at King's College London (KCL) and continuing her academic research in radicalism and terrorism. She has published more than 10 scholarly papers, including "Who is to blame, the victims or the perpetrators?," Coping with stigma and social exclusion of Indonesian terror- convicts' wives," "Tackling Islamic terrorism and radicalism in Indonesia by increasing the sense of humanity & friendship," "Recognition, apology, and restoration of Indonesians' past maltreatment of people labeled as communists," and "Increasing integrative complexity on convicted terrorist in Indonesia."

Joshua Snider is a faculty member at UAE National Defense college in Abu Dhabi. His research focuses on sectarian political violence and terrorism, with a particular focus on Southeast and South Asia. He is particularly interested in violent religiosity in Middle East and South Southeast Asia and how states make and execute P/CVE policy. Prior to arriving in UAE Joshua spent eight years in Malaysia, where he was faculty member in the School of Politics, History and International Relations at the University of Nottingham's Malaysia Campus in Kuala Lumpur. In addition, Joshua has consulted for national governments and international organizations on matters related to CVE program development. Before embarking on an academic career Joshua worked for the Canadian government and in the public affairs consulting industry. He earned his PhD in politics in 2015 from the University of Newcastle, Australia.

Hendro Wibowo completed his Bachelor's degree in Sharia Banking at STEI SEBI, a Master's degree in Sharia Finance at Paramadina University, and his Doctoral dissertation at Asia E University Malaysia. Currently, he is a Lecturer at STEI SEBI and UIN Jakarta. He is active in several organizations, including Deputy Chair of the Central MUI Foreign Cooperation Division; Secretary of the IAEI, MES Central Management; and General Chair of the FoSSEI Alumni Corps. He has won several awards in writing, including First Place in the National Cooperative Economics Essay Competition, Best Paper at the Ministry of National Development Planning/Bappenas, and Best Paper in the National Young Writers Category from the Sharia Banking Research Forum. The books he has been written are *Colors of Islamic Economics, Ferris Wheel of Islamic Economics, Economic Empowerment of Fishermen, Sharia Cooperative Management, What and How to Invest in Hajj Finance, Investment in BPKH Securities*, and *Sharia Capital Markets*.

Thomas Wuchte recently completed his assignment as the Executive Director for the International Institute for Justice and the Rule of Law (IIJ)—leading the intergovernmental organization located in Valletta, Malta. Before the IIJ, he led counterterrorism efforts for the 57 participating states in the Organization for Security and Co-operation in Europe (OSCE) in Vienna, Austria, as the Head of Anti-terrorism. At present, he is the founder of the Center for Multilateral Collaboration and Co-operation Leadership, based in the Washington DC Baltimore area and Bangkok. His focus is on empowering multilateral collaboration on security issues such as climate change—while also working to balance resources for these new issues to better address the conditions conducive to violent extremism and terrorism.

INTRODUCTION

*Rohan Gunaratna, Mohd Mizan Aslam,
and Liu Chunlin*

Introduction

This book offers the best compendium of thematic and countries' perspective on planetary health's strategy post-pandemic COVID-19. Providing a rich array of perspectives on the world's most serious security challenges, scholars, analysts, and practitioners from around the world voice their outlooks through many unique lenses. This book critically analyses the specific security threat posed by COVID-19 to the global society. It offers a comprehensive and critical examination of COVID-19 global responses and challenges, suggesting more balanced and nuanced approaches in establishing the securing a balance planet. Contributors include leading scholars in global security, economics, public health, and information technology as well as social and political activists. These cross-continental experts include renowned world social scientists, as well as highly regarded journalists, academics, medical practitioners, and overall outstanding commentators. This book contains a formidable and unparalleled combination of expertise.

The main focus of the book is on securing our future under planetary health's framework post-pandemic COVID-19. Predominantly, during the formative years of planetary health studies, the discipline was dominated by the singular focus of the causes, challenges and prevention of pandemics. In the name of survival, our ancestors long searched the forest in quest of food and water. Without question, humans and the forest have long had a mutually beneficial connection. However, modern society has undoubtedly taken all of the world's environmental problems—such as the extinction of animal species, rising temperatures, and natural disasters—for granted, even if they are at an all-time high. Many individuals and groups have made efforts to resist such atrocities, but they have tragically been

DOI: 10.4324/9781003569084-1

forgotten as wars are waged and forests destroyed in pursuit of selfish greed and happiness. This goes to show that for a long time we humans have been causing damage to Mother Nature but take little to no heed to the environment, which is ironic because we have benefitted from it all this while. Would it not be fair for us to, at least, try to save it?

Measuring happiness and well-being in any area of daily life is one approach to guarantee the health of the planet in the future. Thus, the idea of integrating security and happiness is presented for the first time in this book. To address global security issues, we are incorporating 'psychology' into security solutions, combining engineering and social science to create comprehensive answers to global security issues. Dr. Chun-lin Liu and Professor Rohan Gunaratna, who authored 'Security & Happiness by Design' (SHBD), are two of the foremost experts in this topic. Dr. Liu first introduced the concept of security and happiness by design in 2008, fine-tuned the methodology alongside Professor Gunaratna in 2022, and has been actively implementing SHBD from 2023 to the present.

The idea of SHBD places a strong emphasis on designing spaces, procedures, and goods that provide equal weight to mental and physical health. It entails creating solutions that not only shield people from harm but also encourage good experiences and raise people's level of enjoyment. By taking proactive steps to address threats beforehand and foster positive experiences, SHBD transforms the conventional framework from a preventive and reactive security mitigation model to one that is centred on creating a user-centric environment with a holistic approach that takes into account both physical and emotional well-being, surrounded by happiness.

SHBD is a new concept for designing and developing security systems that is based on psychology research findings and aims to integrate happiness elements and the complexity of physical safety and protection into the holistic design concept of a facility, starting from the planning stage through the construction and operation phases. The best result is the achievement of security enhancement while balancing ethical considerations, so that SHBD can be implemented in an ethical manner.

Compared to traditional physical crimes, cybercrimes are becoming more common and posing dynamic uncertainties to all security forces because of the increasingly volatile and unpredictable global threat scene, which makes it easy for local conflicts to escalate into larger regional and ultimately global situations. Most of the information infrastructure and vital infrastructure in any country are targets for terrorist and criminal groups. Misinformation, disinformation, and malinformation efforts using cyber tools to instil mistrust, fear, and a host of other emotional negatives are expected to increase.

The physical demarcation of psychological effects at the front lines is no longer valid, and psychological protection is now of utmost importance, particularly in times of peace. By merely concentrating on the understanding of human behaviour and emotions rather than heavily relying on AI technologies to build security solutions that may attract more serious cyber threats, psychological defence through the promotion of SHBD is a novel approach.

In an increasingly interconnected world, the concepts of security and happiness have become pivotal in designing sustainable communities that contribute to a healthy planet. Security, both physical and emotional, lays the foundation for individual and collective well-being. When people feel safe in their environment, they are more likely to engage positively with their community, leading to enhanced social cohesion. This sense of security is critical in addressing global challenges such as climate change, resource scarcity, and socioeconomic disparities. Happiness by design involves creating spaces and systems that enhance well-being through thoughtful planning and policymaking. Urban design, for example, can incorporate green spaces, pedestrian-friendly pathways, and community gardens that foster social interaction and promote mental health. Access to nature not only enhances physical well-being but also provides an escape from the stresses of urban life, fostering a sense of calm and belonging.

Creating a healthy planet necessitates an interdisciplinary approach that integrates environmental stewardship with human-centric design.

Policies encouraging the development of renewable energy sources, sustainable agriculture, and waste management systems promote environmental health while ensuring that communities thrive. This balance of security and happiness cultivates resilience, enabling communities to adapt to changes and challenges. Furthermore, promoting mental and emotional well-being plays a significant role in environmental stewardship. Communities that feel secure and supported are more likely to take collective action for sustainability, participating in initiatives like recycling programs, conservation efforts, and local environmental advocacy.

In conclusion, the synergy of security and happiness by design is essential in creating a healthy planet. By prioritising these principles, we can cultivate environments that not only sustain the planet but also nurture the individuals and communities that inhabit it, ensuring a more sustainable and joyful future for all.

Significance of the Book

Previous approaches to public and global health have traditionally been considered as a focus on the health of people all over the world, with little regard for other natural ecosystems. The *Lancet*, a UK-based medical journal, advocated for collective efforts to modernise the field of public health in 2014, resulting in the notion of planetary health. The concept goes beyond this traditional perspective, becoming an interdisciplinary field of study, addressing several issues such as urbanisation, biodiversity shifts, and the lately alarming issue of food security, and thus deserves much greater attention and action in our daily lives. It emphasises the significance of caring for the health of all systems in our world, whether they be medical, economic, political, or educational. It perceives them as a series of interdependencies that affect the environment and, in turn, us—the people who live on the planet.

A report titled 'Safeguarding human health in the Anthropocene period', issued in 2015 by the Rockefeller Foundation–Lancet Commission on Planetary Health, resulted in the founding of the Planetary Health Alliance, an organisation dedicated to addressing the challenges mentioned in the report. As pioneers in this endeavour, the alliance brings together hundreds of organisations to lead activities in planetary health research and education. Through this collaboration, it hopes to prepare the community towards the 'Great Transition', redefining how we interact with each other and the nature.

In order to improve planetary health, it encourages active collaboration among professionals from many sectors as well as international institutions such as multinational corporations, governments, and their labour unions. However, planetary health should not be considered solely as a concern for major organisations to solve, since every individuals can play a role in matters as simple as practising the 3Rs as a regular routine. It is apparent that planetary health has a far greater impact on our lives than we realise. As a result, its significance can be separated into three broad categories: importance to individuals, businesses, and the government. In terms of individuals, planetary health has a significant impact on our health, primarily through attempts to mitigate climate change as well as protecting natural resources essential for survival (i.e., food and water supply).

When businesses apply sustainable practices, such as the UN's proposed Sustainable Development Goals (SDGs) and Environmental, Social, and Governance (ESG) principles, the production of goods and services is more likely to cause less environmental harm and result in a much healthier lifestyle, giving them higher credibility for their corporate social responsibility (CSR) efforts. State entities would certainly fulfil their responsibilities by enacting policies that encourage such practices, and in return benefit from the innovation and investment opportunities. Planetary health clearly demands a paradigm shift in how we think about ties between state and non-state actors, as each policy, corporate agreement, and even educational system will have a significant impact on our daily lives. Simply said, planetary health is an effort to stabilise our planet's life-support systems, resulting in a self-sustaining system revolving around us.

Although achieving planetary health has many advantages, it faces numerous problems in achieving its objectives. The first challenge, and arguably the most difficult, would be to collaborate across sectors. This is consistent with the prevailing norm of putting short-term personal welfare ahead of long-term community welfare. A good example would be in the case of illegal logging. Studies have shown that illegal logging is not purely a choice by individuals but a consequence of working systems, be it legal or illegal, encouraging such practice. Factors such as the laxity of forest protection laws and rural poverty makes the black market much more attractive, as the same resources can be obtained at much cheaper prices. This in turn, affects not only countries permitting such activity but everyone since it affects the global economy through lowered timber prices that risk future price soars caused by scarcity. To tackle the problem, we must look beyond the tip of the iceberg. In this scenario, it would be to acknowledge that, despite the many protests and educational attempts at discouraging illegal logging, there must be reasons for the expanding practice of illegal logging. As a result, it is necessary to establish the interdependence between survival for short-term well-being and long-term well-being for the community. Root problems could be found to be a lack of infrastructure, the development of a significant shadow economy, or even corruption from those in power, making law enforcement merely a temporary deterrent.

Another challenge in planetary health is the rapidly changing and unstable ecological and geopolitical context, which necessitates timely and decisive intervention. Issues such as the continuing Ukraine–Russia war and the Yemeni civil war make efforts to implement planetary health much more difficult. These disagreements limit opportunities to educate about the critical issue of our planet's health, leaving future generations unprepared for the Great Transition. The lack of a government committed to such goals makes domestic administration of sustainable practices difficult, not to mention limiting opportunities for international collaboration. As a result, the subject of global security must not be treated lightly, especially now that planetary frailness is imminent due to the huge impediments that it creates.

Finally, there is a paucity of research and information on applying sustainable practices around the world. It must be recognised that each country suffers its own unique obstacles, such as the lack of infrastructure or food shortages. As a result, governments cannot afford to merely replicate a blueprint for sustainable operations and must instead adapt with their resources at hand. However, the distinction between adapting and compromising must be highlighted. It is necessary to innovate on sustainable practices, but this cannot be taken for granted merely because it cannot be 'afforded'. This leads back to the need for collective efforts across borders to provide mentorship and guidance towards building each country its own version of a planetary health system. This calls for more organisations to be formed with the same vision as the public health authority (PHA), as this is no longer a national issue but a planetary issue, and thus requires setting aside political differences and welcoming assistance. We have long harmed our global ecology, and now is the time to make a difference.

Chapters

This book starts with Chapter One on the importance of planetary health after the COVID-19 Pandemic, in which Professor Aslam discusses the concept planetary health. It starts with 'individual health' revolving around the human being. However, 'public health' emphasises the connectivity among people in society and how secure healthcare is a product of collective effort rather than an individual accomplishment, especially fighting against the transmission of infectious diseases. On the other hand, 'global heath' goes beyond the collective responsibility of healthcare and highlights that socioeconomic factors play a major role in establishing secure health systems. As a result, it showcases the nexus between money and advanced health practices/systems. Then, 'one health' portrays the connectivity of wildlife and natural living elements to the health of the individuals. Beyond that, planetary health has been discussed as a mechanism which 'recognises the health of the planet as a system, and that even its non-living components are wrapped up in that state of well-being or disease'. In 2015 *The Lancet* medical journal and Rockefeller Foundation jointly published a report which emphasised that human beings have harmed the natural systems of the planet, which now backlashes at the health of the humans. The report further emphasised that there is a need for adjusting the existing mechanisms which damage the natural systems in the Earth. It urged a collective international approach in restoring the natural functions of the planet we live on today ensuring planetary health, which reciprocates the health of the human being by reducing the spread of diseases. Within such context, planetary health has become a vital component in the post-pandemic health system due to its holistic approach towards the well-being of the individual and due to the correlation of how natural systems influence the health of human beings in a rapidly changing environment. As a result, the post-pandemic context has emphasised the importance of indigenous medicine, which connects with nature and also makes human beings close to the natural systems which enhance healthcare.

Muhd Nabhan Mizan in Chapter Two discusses the global perspective of planetary health. Nabhan gives a viewpoint of planetary health that encourages individuals and organisations at any level or in any field to observe the bigger picture. It does not require the complete overhaul of existing systems; instead, it builds upon them and encourages us to understand their interconnections. Consequently, it bridges the gap between experts and users in various fields. This now entails new sets of challenges, such as coming to a common consensus among the many stakeholders. It now competes among the many other issues faced by these stakeholders, addressing the question of saliency and understanding how hard it is to implement at the local and, even more so, at the international level. The shift of focus towards protecting the world against climate change has long been discussed, and green efforts are now taking centre stage more than ever before. So, the question now is, Why should planetary health be discussed? For a long period of time, we have viewed public health through the traditional lens of medicine and public health as a niche study that is exclusive to doctors, scientists, and physicists alike. However, approaching public health through such siloed views threatens the effectiveness of public health efforts as there is a lack of inclusivity and exchange of ideas among specialists in different fields. It is often enough that public health concerns are unheard of or dismissed at policy levels of implementation.

In Chapter Three, John Harrison and Immanuel Azzad discusses the Western commitment to planetary health. After the Rockefeller Foundation–Lancet Commission Report was published in 2015, it inspired the creation of a new academic field called planetary health, as a reaction to the world's ongoing environmental problems and crises (Whitmee et al., 2015). Medical ecologists established this field decades ago, and Indigenous societies have long held the belief that human health and the natural environment are interwoven, as do medical ecologists. The growth of planetary health as an academic effort, as a result, acts as an umbrella to bring scientists and politicians together around a common issue and influences research agendas advocated by varied alliances. As a result of this deliberate effort to include opinions from a diverse range of scientific domains, experts from various disciplines can lend their support to the project. It is a top goal for practitioners to understand how social systems influence the planet's health, and social scientists are invited to contribute to this understanding (Iyers, 2021). To ensure global well-being, it is necessary to do in-depth research into the relationship between human economic activity and the evolution of the Earth's systems. It is feasible to find solutions to problems that appear intractable from a single scientific area perspective. When evidence from a range of disciplines is used to support a policy, the case for the policy becomes more powerful.

Joshua Snider examined the COVID-19 in the Himalayan region: state capacity and non-traditional security challenges in Chapter Four. The COVID-19 pandemic is without question the most significant and most severe global public health crisis in the past century. The depth and severity of the crisis can be understood at the inter-state and intra-state levels. At the inter-state level, pandemic-driven border closures disrupted tourism travel trade, which has had knock-on effects at the sub-state level in terms of food, energy, and societal security. At the intra-state level, the pandemic's toll can be measured by the loss of life, the impact on public health systems, and disruptions to education and the economy. The pandemic was a perfect storm for lower- and middle-income states generally. In the Indo-Pacific region, dynamics such as low state capacity, weak and under-funded public health systems, limited social welfare programs, ethno-religious populism, and low trust in governments, combined with demographic factors such as high-density living, multi-generational families, and transient and mobile populations all conspired to create an uncontrollable situation with respect to the states' governance of the COVID-19 pandemic. Amidst the pandemic's catastrophic impact on large states in the Indo-Pacific, there has been comparatively little focus on the pandemic's impact on smaller states and sub-regions. Moreover, the economic precarity of large peasant populations reliant on subsistence wages meant that states did not have the option to enact long-term lockdowns, nor did they have the resources to keep large and vulnerable populations out of poverty. Indeed, pandemic-driven precarity will be a structural challenge for lower- and middle-income states across the Indo-Pacific for decades to come.

In Chapter Five, Liu Chunlin and Rohan Gunaratna discuss the global pandemic's impact: the shift from the physical to online and hybrid domains. Liu and Rohan explain how the natural and human-made disasters threaten planetary health. The intermittent shocks the planet suffered – such as the most recent COVID-19 pandemic – disrupted society. The pandemic's profound impact limited face-to-face human interaction and created a hybrid environment. Unless humanity respects nature and planetary health is maintained, society will suffer such shocks more frequently, to the point of overwhelming humanity. Until a code of ethics and a set of values govern humanity to reinforce planetary health, we will live in a compromised world. The focus of the chapter is on the changed security landscape from the physical to the digital. The new normal, the hybrid environment, has profound implications for security. All security assessments in future will have to consider the implications of the pandemic and the post-pandemic world. Today, most company data is stored in the cloud or in the company server accessed by the internet. Most staff share office facilities, and many offices have shared tables. The paperless office is the norm. Furthermore, people's behaviour has changed. Rather than meeting physically, they meet virtually. Virtual interaction – deemed more efficient – saves time and cost. Are there limitations to the expanding virtual living? Physical interaction is still important to understand each other better. The human experience of consciousness is a mere epiphenomenon of cerebral biochemistry. To build relationships and trust, we must meet physically. Some problems cannot be effectively resolved through virtual interfacing. As some relationships are hard to build and sustain virtually, physical interfacing is imperative. As such, the new security paradigm should consider both the physical and virtual dimensions.

Kyounggon Kim, in Chapter Six, examines planetary health in cybersecurity and cybercrime in the Middle East. The Middle East and North Africa (MENA) region is a very important region that is connected to three continents: Africa, Asia, and Europe. The MENA region is currently moving towards a digital society more than at any other time in history. The world has inevitably demanded a change to a digital society according to the changes of the times. However, even though the change to a digital society has many advantages, new threats to countries, companies, and individuals, such as cybercrime and cyberattacks, arise. In this chapter, our proposal focuses on cooperation, capability, and assessment (CCA) for cybersecurity and cybercrime in the MENA region. We hope that these important factors will help maintain the ongoing cybersecurity and international peace of the MENA.

In Chapter Seven, Thomas Wuchte discusses the policy implications of climate change and violent extremism in global perspectives. One would hope that the better part of humanity would have come out the other side of the COVID-19 pandemic with a renewed sense of purpose – tackling such challenges as this climate change, lifting poverty conditions within developing countries, solving water deficits, and forming collective approaches to the loss of natural habitat for species other than humankind. As young diplomats, many sat transfixed by the burning twin towers and today recall thinking to one another: 'This is bad, but we can't overreact, or we will squander the international goodwill'. The past several years have added fuel to some of the decisions we made in the responses to terrorism and COVID-19 which empowered uninterrupted 'stay-at-home' time to receive excellent disinformation that fuels current disagreements in politics. The nexus of these concerns and climate change takes the view that we can and should move beyond calls to understand the linkages between the effects of climate change and the risks of recruitment to violent extremism – the past 20 years are replete with evidence by a large cadre of experts and data and studies that can point to such linkages that we have had presented as the counterterrorism architecture has grown.[1] Violent extremist groups will leverage governance failures to increase the effects of climate change. How to respond is about elevating this as a threat to peace and security with a similar consensus within the United Nations (these thoughts were developed at the high-level UN General Assembly week 2023) and cascading downwards to regional organisations and then national priorities.

A country perspective is deliberated by Any Rufaedah in Chapter Eight, discussing the recovery strategy: the efforts of East Timor government in resolving crisis. Four years after its formal independence, East Timor (Timor-Leste) was stormed by open clashes involving two ethnonational groups: Loromonu (westerners) and Lorosae (easterners) in 2006. The clashes started from a petition from Loromonu military officers (petitioners) complaining about perceived discrimination against them. The clashes dragged the country to a crisis, resulting in up to 38 deaths, more than 100,000 internally displaced persons (IDPs), and thousands of houses destroyed. The crisis continued for at least two years, to 2008. Further attacks and violence carried out by a rebel group, gangs, and martial art groups reportedly occurred; in addition approximately 30,000 IDPs remained in camps and 70,000 in the house of families or friends. This chapter explores factors behind the crisis, efforts of the East Timor government to overcome the crisis, and current updates on the security sector. Studies found multiple factors triggering the crisis, including perceived discrimination from westerners to easterners in the military force and police department, political rivalry, economic and educational gap, weakness of national identity, and fault in the police recruitment process. Some officials in the defence department were proven to have been involved in distributing weapons to rebels. In response to the crisis, the government, with the assistance of international communities, created strategies that focused on security reform, IDPs, and compensation for former pro-East Timor militias and rebels. The strategies were considered effective to halt further violence, proven by the absence of similar violence. Nonetheless, clashes between martial groups and conflicts for land remain.

Lihini Ratwatte's chapter titled 'The Gendered Impact of Crises: Operationalising Sri Lanka's Women, Peace and Security Agenda for Recovery and Regeneration' is presented in Chapter Nine. The gendered impact of crises highlights the changing nature of peace and security while reiterating the urgency for women's engagement in leadership and peacebuilding. This chapter views COVID-19[2] as 'mimicking' conflict-like dynamics due to emergency powers and militarised directives being used to mitigate response and recovery efforts. With key references to Sri Lanka and parallels drawn from the South Asian region, the chapter highlights how crises can exacerbate existing gender inequalities and disproportionately affect women by hindering their meaningful participation in leadership, their economic empowerment and personal safety. Against this back-drop, the chapter underlines how Sri Lanka is in a unique position to operation-alise its National Action Plan on Women, Peace and Security towards recovery and regeneration. With close reference to the foundations laid out in UN Security Council Resolution 1325 on Women, Peace and Security (UNSCR 1325), the chapter utilises an intersectional lens to identify how women can become cata-lysts of peace, whilst being at the forefront of recovery and regeneration within a post–COVID-19 era. The chapter deconstructs the theoretical premise presented by the 'Regenerative State', which makes a case for the state to address gender disparities when developing inclusive policies aimed at socioeconomic recovery, as it brings alternative responses to the table and ensures gender sensitive protec-tions for all. The key findings of the chapter attest that a holistic Women, Peace and Security agenda recognises women's meaningful leadership in recovery as a 'rights-based' approach.

In the final chapter, Efri Syamsul Bahri, Hendro Wibowo, Pamungkas Hen-dra Kusuma, and Nur Efendi examine the Islamic Social Finance Contribution in Pandemic COVID-19: Evidence From Indonesia. The research results by Susila-wati et al. (2020) illustrate that the COVID-19 pandemic affected the Indonesian economy. Susilawati et al. (2020) describe several sectors affected by COVID-19, including transportation, tourism, and trade. However, the economic sector was considerably affected by COVID-19, especially household economies. Fitri-ani (2020) finds that stopping economic activity affects income. Fitriani (2020) mentions that the impact of the COVID-19 pandemic is the loss of employment, which affects vulnerable groups. Mustahiq is an element of the society affected by COVID-19. According to Fitriani (2020), people were unable to meet their daily needs because they lost their income. Fitriani (2020) classified mustahiq affected by the COVID-19 pandemic into vulnerable groups, small and medium business groups, and groups with disabilities. Islamic social finance played a strategic role in overcoming the mustahiq's burden. In Indonesia, Islamic social finance collects and distributes funds sourced from Islamic social finance, namely, zakat, infaq/alm, waqf, and humanitarian donations. Olanrewaju et al. (2020) explain that Islamic social finance, which comes from zakat, infaq/alms, and waqf, is an Islamic system that represents a robust socioeconomic structure that redistributes wealth to reduce poverty in society. In a recent article concludes that Islamic social finance could be an explanation for handling COVID-19 consequences by using zakat, donations, and alms to meet consumptive needs and endowments used in health infrastructure assistance. This analysis is in line with that of Rizal and Mukaromah (2020), who state that zakat, infaq/alms, and waqf funds can increase purchasing power and overcome poverty.

Conclusion

In conclusion, this book is a valuable and rich collection on global COVID-19 response towards planetary health. The multitude of challenges can be seen through the examples in the chapters of this book. The empirical evidence attached to the various case studies covers global perspectives on COVID-19 response. Various experiences and practices aligning with strengths and weaknesses in tackling unprecedented modern history of pandemic issues are discussed thoroughly. It is important to have a clear sight and understanding of the challenges in engaging the issues of COVID-19 in order to create a balanced and healthy lifestyle. The book consists of ten chapters with an array of discussions on COVID-19 response to major sectors, which are security, defence, trade, economy, health, digital, religion, and community.

This book can be used as recommended reading for a course in an academic institute or a policy-oriented class. The edited volume could be assigned as core reading material for undergraduate and post-graduate courses and modules. In addition, it can be used as a reference for academic studies and research. The country case studies within the book are intended to provide a guide for policy makers, ministries, and law enforcement agencies in developing the best functional post–COVID-19 response. This book is also relevant for online and offline conference proceedings; it can be used as a guide for policymakers and governments who are looking to understand best practices from all around the world in response to the pandemic.

Notes

1 See, for example, Bourekba M. (2021) 'Climate Change and Violent Extremism in North Africa'. Barcelona Centre for International Affairs (CIDOB), pages 15–16, as well as material published on this topic with the US Institute of Peace (USIP). You can find the USIP brief here, which notes that the US Department of Defense has longstanding efforts on the impact of changing climate conditions on defence infrastructure and the operating environment: Burke S. (2023) 'Achieving Climate Security'.
2 Authors note: As the chapter was sent for publication in 2021, the author has only viewed 'COVID-19' as a crisis mimicking conflict-like dynamics. In this chapter, the author has not considered Sri Lanka's political and economic crisis that ensued in 2022. The author acknowledges that the events surrounding 2022 can add more nuance to the arguments presented in this chapter and continues her research on how the women, peace and security agenda can respond to Sri Lanka's 'converging crises'.

References

Fitriani, F. (2020). *Women's empowerment and economic growth in rural Indonesia.* United Nations Development Programme. https://www.undp.org

Rizal, A., & Mukaromah, M. (2020). *Digital innovation and entrepreneurship in Indonesia.* Springer.

Susilawati, S., Smith, J., & Johnson, L. (2020). *Climate resilience in agriculture: Case studies from Southeast Asia.* Springer.

Whitmee, S., Haines, A., Beyrer, C., Boltz, F., Capon, A. G., de Souza Dias, B. F., Ezeh, A., Frumkin, H., Gong, P., Head, P., Horton, R., Mace, G. M., Marten, R., Myers, S. S., Nishtar, S., Osofsky, S. A., Pattanayak, S. K., Pongsiri, M. J., Romanelli, C., ... Yach, D. (2015). Safeguarding human health in the Anthropocene epoch: Report of The Rockefeller Foundation–Lancet Commission on planetary health. *The Lancet, 386*(10007), 1973–2028. https://doi.org/10.1016/S0140-6736(15)60901-1

1

THE IMPORTANCE OF PLANETARY HEALTH AFTER THE COVID-19 PANDEMIC

Mohd Mizan Aslam

1.1 Introduction

The COVID-19 pandemic, which started in December 2019 from Wuhan in China, emphasised the weak health care systems, social inequalities, and socio-economic instabilities around the world. Irrespective of whether countries are rich or poor, developed or developing, all have been affected by the pandemic, challenging the existing governing structures and systems, particularly in terms of health care arrangements. As a result, during the post-pandemic era, the description of 'health' has been extended from 'individual health care' to 'planetary health' due to the correlation between the security of the individual and well-being of the planet. Therefore, the health of the individual is linked to the well-being of the planet and vice versa. Hence, health care has taken a more holistic approach not only focusing on the individual but also discussing how the well-being of the planet is ensuring prosperous health systems to the individual.

The COVID-19 pandemic that raged across the whole world in December 2019 has not only exposed the vulnerability of global health care systems but has also brought attention to broader issues of social inequality and socioeconomic volatility. Regardless of their status or level of development, countries worldwide have been impacted by the pandemic, prompting a reassessment of existing governance structures and health care systems. As a result, the concept of health has emerged, recognising the inherent correlation between individual health and the well-being of our planet.

The concept of 'individual health' revolves around the human being. However, 'public health' emphasises the connectivity between people in society and how secure health care is a product of collective effort rather than an individual accomplishment, especially fighting against transmission of infectious diseases. On

DOI: 10.4324/9781003569084-2

the other hand, 'global heath' goes beyond the collective responsibility of health care and highlights that socioeconomic factors play a major role in establishing secure health systems. As a result, it showcases the nexus between money and advanced health practices/systems. Then, one health portrays the connectivity of wildlife and natural living elements to the health of the individuals. Beyond that, planetary health has been discussed as a mechanism which 'recognises the health of the planet as a system, and that even its non-living components are wrapped up in that state of well-being or disease.' Whitmee et al., 2015.

In 2015 the *Lancet* medical journal and Rockefeller Foundation conjointly published a report that emphasised that human beings have harmed the natural systems of the planet, which now have a backlash effect on the health of the humans. The report further emphasised that there is a need for adjusting the existing mechanisms which damage the natural systems in the earth. It urged a collective international approach in restoring the natural functions of the planet we live in today, ensuring planetary health which reciprocates the health of the human being by reducing spread of diseases. Within such a context, planetary health has become a vital component in the post-pandemic health system due to its holistic approach towards the well-being of the individual and due to the correlation of how natural systems influence the health of the human beings in a rapidly changing environment. As a result, the post-pandemic context has emphasised the importance of indigenous medicine, which connects with the nature and also brings human beings close to the natural systems, which enhances health care.

At the same time, the pandemic was a wake-up call for all humans, making them understand that human beings are part of the natural system but are not the driving forces of the system. Before the pandemic, humans behaved as if they owned the entire plant, while utilising its resources for their own advantage, forgetting that they are part of a system. However, with the pandemic it became evident that the health systems that were in place were not adequate to face such a situation since the system did not see planetary health and its influence on individual health as a major component. The focus was mostly on individual health or public health, without going beyond and experiencing how natural systems are a part of human well-being.

Therefore, the COVID-19 pandemic emphasised the importance of

- Reinforcing climate resilience in economies and ecosystems while promoting conjunction of climate, biodiversity, and health finance
- Establishing economies with resource efficiency and ecosystem-based approach
- Financially assisting biodiversity and ecosystem protection to avoid eruptions of infectious diseases and fortify nutritional security
- Reconstructing data patterns at all levels, including interdisciplinary and coinciding risk dynamics
- Establishing a multi-sectorial and multidisciplinary approach in health care systems.

- Encouraging policy orientation in international/intergovernmental/regional and national organisations to promote planetary health for a sustainable health care system in each and every country in the world

1.2   Planetary Health Definitions

Planetary health is a worldwide movement, a new science for extraordinary action, and a paradigm for multidisciplinary and transdisciplinary study. 'The health of human civilisation and the state of the natural systems on which it depends' is what is meant by planetary health. The idea for a new health science with more than 25 areas of competence was introduced by the Rockefeller Foundation–Lancet Commission on Planetary Health in 2015.

A planetary health perspective to human development acknowledges that, as seen by the industrial, green, and technological revolutions, humanity has advanced significantly in many areas. However, the planet's health is now being clearly disrupted, offsetting these development gains. Depleted biodiversity, shifting land use and cover, a sharp rise in air pollution, a lack of natural resources, and the harm these factors cause to our living environment are all examples of this, as seen by recent pandemics, disease outbreaks, and the climate emergency. A transdisciplinary, solutions-oriented field and social movement, planetary health examines and resolves the effects of human disturbances of Earth's natural systems on human health and all life on the planet.

Planetary health is a recent term that is premised on the notion that human well-being in the long term is dependent on the well-being of the Earth, including living and non-living systems. Formally, planetary health has been defined as 'the health of human civilization and the natural systems on which it depends'. It is an interdisciplinary field whose principal aim is to characterise and quantify the impacts of human-mediated disruptions of the Earth resources and systems on human health. According to the Rockefeller Foundation–Lancet Commission on Planetary Health, human health and the health of our planet are closely intertwined, and the well-being of people, healthy natural systems, and prudent use of natural resources are all essential to our civilisation. Our health and the health of our world are in danger due to the enormous degradation of natural systems.

Planetary health is defined as the health of human populations and the state of the natural systems on which it depends. Urgent attention and action is required to address the extensive damage that humans have created and acknowledge our health is intrinsically linked to the health of the planet. The Rockefeller Foundation–Lancet Commission on Planetary Health defined planetary health as the health of human civilisations and the natural systems on which they depend. To explain this idea in simpler terms we need to think of human beings as a powerful and growing force behind the environmental change that we are witnessing today. Alterations to climate, water, land, and ecosystems are challenging all life on our planet, with serious implications for human health. The way we think about the planet needs to be revised, as does the approach we take in interacting with it.

The study of the relationships between human health and the health of the living and non-living ecosystems that support human life on Earth is known as planetary health. Planetary health is based on the idea that the long-term health of humans is reliant on the health of the world, including its living and non-living systems. According to the panel, humankind is in better health than it has ever been—at least before the COVID-19 pandemic. Life expectancy has increased. Poverty has decreased. Child mortality has decreased. However, these developments have resulted in the overuse of natural resources, many of which are non-renewable and others that replenish over periods of time that are significantly faster than the rates at which they are being used in the Anthropocene.

Planetary health is an emerging trans-disciplinary field, encompassing the connections between human health and the natural/physical sciences, and broadly integrating the related fields of public health, geo health, one health, global health, etc. A complicated field, planetary health is, perhaps, best defined by the Rockefeller–Lancet Commission in its 2015 report as 'the health of human civilization and the state of the natural systems on which it depends'.

1.3 Countries That Have Implemented Planetary Health

Delving into planetary health initiatives in Bhutan, Sweden, Costa Rica, and New Zealand offers a fascinating insight into how these countries are leading the charge towards a more sustainable and interconnected future. Let's explore each country's unique approach in further detail.

1.3.1 Bhutan

Bhutan, renowned for its focus on gross national happiness, has integrated planetary health into its policymaking. With a deep-rooted reverence for nature, Bhutan boasts a remarkably high forest cover, helping sequester carbon and preserve biodiversity. The country prioritises renewable energy sources, such as hydroelectric power, to reduce reliance on fossil fuels. By emphasising sustainable practices like organic agriculture and ecotourism, Bhutan showcases a holistic approach to planetary health that intertwines environmental conservation with societal well-being.

1.3.2 Sweden

Sweden stands out for its proactive stance on sustainability and environmental stewardship. The nation has set ambitious targets for transitioning to a low-carbon economy, embracing renewable energy sources like wind and solar power. Sweden's sustainable urban planning focuses on reducing emissions and creating green spaces for its citizens. The Swedish government's commitment to sustainability is evident in policies promoting recycling, sustainable transportation, and initiatives to mitigate climate change. By prioritising sustainable development and innovation, Sweden serves as a model for planetary health initiatives on a global scale.

1.3.3　Costa Rica

Costa Rica's rich biodiversity and conservation efforts exemplify its dedication to planetary health. The country aims to be carbon-neutral by 2050, leveraging its natural resources to drive sustainable practices. Costa Rica champions renewable energy, with a significant portion of its electricity derived from sources like hydropower and geothermal energy. Conservation efforts, such as reforestation projects and protected areas, contribute to the nation's commitment to preserving its natural habitats. Costa Rica's emphasis on eco-tourism and sustainable agriculture underscores its holistic approach to planetary health, blending environmental conservation with economic prosperity.

1.3.4　New Zealand

New Zealand's focus on well-being and sustainability underscores its planetary health initiatives. The country's well-being budget prioritises the holistic health of its citizens, emphasising mental health, social connectedness, and environmental sustainability. New Zealand has taken significant steps to address climate change, setting targets to reduce greenhouse gas emissions and promote renewable energy sources. The nation's commitment to conservation is evident in initiatives to protect its unique biodiversity and natural landscapes. By integrating planetary health principles into its policymaking, New Zealand showcases a comprehensive approach to sustainable development that balances economic prosperity with environmental preservation.

In conclusion, Bhutan, Sweden, Costa Rica, and New Zealand exemplify the diverse strategies and approaches to planetary health implemented by different countries. Despite their unique contexts, these nations share a common goal of fostering sustainable development, environmental stewardship, and societal well-being. By learning from the successes and challenges of these countries, we can collectively work towards a healthier and more resilient future for both humanity and the planet.

1.4　Understanding Planetary Health

The notion of health encompasses a perspective that acknowledges the interdependence between human well-being and environmental health (Whitmee et al., 2015). It centres around recognising that individuals' security and welfare are intricately tied to the well-being of our planet. This viewpoint highlights the significance of the environment in preserving human health. Recently, there has been a growing focus on health, which recognises the direct impact of environmental challenges such as pollution, climate change, and habitat destruction on human well-being (Whitmee et al., 2015).

For instance, respiratory illnesses have been linked to air pollution (Haines et al., 2015). Extreme weather events exacerbated by climate change can have public health implications (Watts et al., 2015). Loss of biodiversity can also disrupt ecosystems, affecting the availability of food and resources while increasing disease risks (Di Marco et al., 2019; Mirza & Rauhala, 2021). These findings highlight the need to address environmental concerns for the sake of public health. The COVID-19 pandemic has underscored the link between health and the well-being of the planet (Wilcox et al., 2019). Diseases, like COVID-19, potentially originating from animals and spreading to humans, serve as a reminder of the importance of preserving biodiversity and ecosystems.

Deforestation, the destruction of habitats, and the illegal wildlife trade can increase the odds of transmitting zoonotic diseases (Wilcox et al., 2019). This shows that efforts aimed at preserving ecosystems and biodiversity play a role in preventing future pandemics and safeguarding human health.

1.5 Importance of Comprehensive Policies and Governance

Governments and international organizations have a role to play in promoting the welfare of society by implementing policies and governing frameworks (IPCC, 2018; United Nations, 2015). Collaborative endeavours such as the Paris Agreement aim to tackle climate change by limiting the increase in temperature to less than 2 degrees Celsius above pre-industrial levels, with an even more ambitious target of 1.5 degrees Celsius. The United Nations Sustainable Development Goals, which are part of the 2030 Agenda for Sustainable Development, cover environmental issues that are crucial for enhancing well-being worldwide. These initiatives align with the principles of well-being by providing a framework for addressing climate change and sustainable development—both components of promoting overall well-being.

In light of COVID-19 an opportunity arises to adopt a more comprehensive and sustainable approach to health care. Planetary health recognises the interconnectedness between well-being and the health of our planet, offering a forward-thinking solution (Willetts & de Paula, 2023). By prioritising health, we can build resilient and equitable health care systems that benefit both people and our planet. This approach aligns with the advocacy for a perspective known as 'one health', which emphasises the interconnectedness of animal and environmental health (Zinsstag et al., 2011).

1.6 Benefits of Prioritising Planetary Health

Prioritising planetary health brings advantages, including better public health outcomes (Myers, 2017). It can also enhance our ability to tackle pandemics by addressing the underlying environmental factors that contribute to disease emergence (Myers, 2017). Additionally, prioritising planetary health promotes a shift towards prevention than just treatment encouraging healthier lifestyles and sustainable practices (Myers, 2017). This aligns with the principles of health and preventive medicine which highlight the importance of addressing root causes for overall improvement in health and well-being (Willetts & de Paula, 2023).

The concept of individual health revolves around the human being. However, public health emphasises the connectivity between people in society and how secure health care is a product of collective effort rather than an individual accomplishment, especially fighting against transmission of infectious diseases. On the other hand, 'global heath' goes beyond the collective responsibility of health care and highlights that socioeconomic factors play a major role in establishing secure health systems. As a result, it showcases the nexus between money and advanced health practices/systems. Then, one health portrays the connectivity of wildlife and natural living elements to the health of the individuals. Beyond that, planetary health has been discussed as a mechanism which 'recognises the health of the planet as a system, and that even its non-living components are wrapped up in that state of well-being or disease'. (Drake, 2021). See the Introduction to this chapter for information on the Rockefeller–Lancet report on the integration of natural and human systems.

During the post-pandemic situation, certain countries have shown interest and commitment towards enhancing 'planetary health.' Particularly, Malaysia is considered the first country in Southeast Asia to implement initiatives aligning to the improvement of planetary health (Mahmood, 2023). Malaysia has initiated a plan that covers the entire nation to 'address ecosystems, biodiversity, health, and climate change in the push to achieve truly people- and planet-centric development' (Mahmood, 2023). This 'whole of nation' approach was implemented in 2024. This approach also favours Prime Minister Datuk Seri Anwar Ibrahim's governing vision of 'Malaysia Madani'. The word 'madani' stands for six core values: 'sustainability, prosperity, innovation, respect, trust, and compassion' (Mahmood, 2023). It is said that Malaysia is projecting towards economic growth through sustainable development while preserving the natural ecosystems in its country.

Following in the footprints of Malaysia, President Joko Widodo of Indonesia is also looking at improving global health care systems through sustainable means in the post-pandemic context. As the chair of the G20, Indonesia is focusing on '[g]lobal health resilience which needs to be viewed beyond the traditional focus on health-care systems and instead, encompass the resilience of human societies and the natural ecosystems on which their health depends' (Mahmood & Guinto, 2022). Consequently, the countries in Southeast Asia are focusing more on the planetary health as a means to improving health care systems in the post-pandemic era, since they have realised that the existing systems are lacking in fulfilling the needs of a global health crisis such as COVID-19.

On the other hand, many of the global players in health care, such as United States of America, Australia, United Kingdom, India, and countries in the Global

South, are yet to see planetary health as a mechanism or a solution for improving the health care systems. That is not to emphasise that such countries have neglected the phenomenon, but mostly they have coupled planetary health with the sustainable development goals, which align with climate change, creating sustainable economies, etc. Therefore, the policies and strategies are associated with the sustainable development goals, not distinctly concentrating on planetary health. However, there is also a significant aspect of economic development clashing with planetary health, and as a result, the countries are also in a dilemma of balancing economic growth and the well-being of the planet (Mukherjee, 2021). That can be a reason why planetary health is often seen as a part of sustainable development. *Having said that, planetary health is yet to be seen as a separate phenomenon which aligns with the health care systems of the countries in the world.*

In conclusion, emphasis on planetary health has become a significant aspect in the health care system during the post-pandemic situation. Many countries in Southeast Asia, such as Malaysia and Indonesia, have realised the importance focusing on planetary health to improve the health care systems while treating the phenomena as a separate element. 'The Kuala Lumpur Declaration on Planetary Health' encourages universities and individuals to implement practices that promote sustainable development and to generate research on planetary health (Withers et al., 2020). However, the entire world has yet to see the importance to focusing on planetary health as a separate element, especially in improving the health care systems, since mostly it is treated as a part of a component aligning to sustainable development goals. Even if planetary health is part of sustainable development goals, when articulating policies it should be treated as a separate aspect, rather than blending it with poverty, climate change, or any other aspect. Hence, this paper emphasises the importance of planetary health during the post-pandemic situation and its importance in improving the health care systems in the world.

1.7   The Importance of Planetary Health

Planetary health is a concept that highlights the connection between the health of the environment and the health of human populations. It recognises that the well-being of people is intimately linked to the well-being of the planet as a whole (Centers for Disease Control and Prevention, 2022). This interconnectedness is crucial to understand as we face pressing global challenges such as climate change, biodiversity loss, and emerging infectious diseases.

To truly grasp the importance of planetary health, it is essential to recognise the intricate web of relationships that exist between human health and the health of the planet. Our actions as individuals, communities, and societies have far-reaching consequences on the environment, which in turn impact our health and well-being. This recognition calls for a shift towards a more holistic and sustainable approach to managing our natural resources and ecosystems.

One key aspect of planetary health is the recognition of the impact of environmental degradation on human health. Pollution, deforestation, climate change, and loss of biodiversity all have direct and indirect effects on human health. For example, air pollution from fossil fuel combustion can lead to respiratory problems, cardiovascular diseases, and even premature death. Deforestation contributes to habitat destruction and loss of biodiversity, which can increase the risk of zoonotic diseases jumping from animals to humans.

Furthermore, climate change poses a significant threat to both human health and the environment. Rising global temperatures can lead to more frequent and more severe natural disasters such as hurricanes, droughts, and wildfires, which have devastating effects on human populations (Nagarik Network, 2020). In addition, changes in climate patterns can alter the distribution of disease vectors such as mosquitoes, leading to the spread of diseases like malaria and dengue fever into new regions.

Protecting planetary health is not just a matter of environmental conservation; it is also essential for ensuring social and economic well-being. Healthy ecosystems provide essential services to human societies, such as clean water, fertile soil, and pollination of crops. By protecting and restoring these ecosystems, we can safeguard our own health and prosperity for future generations.

In conclusion, planetary health is a critically important concept that emphasises the interconnectedness of human health and the health of the planet. By recognising and addressing the environmental challenges we face, we can create a more sustainable and resilient future for both people and the planet. It is imperative that we take action now to protect and preserve our natural environment for the well-being of current and future generations.

1.7.1   Understanding Consequences of Planetary Health

Understanding the consequences of planetary health is crucial in order to grasp the full impact of environmental degradation on human well-being, social structures, economies, and ecosystems. The concept of planetary health emphasises the interconnectedness of environmental sustainability and human health, highlighting the fact that our actions as a species have far-reaching consequences for the health of the planet as a whole.

One of the most immediate and tangible consequences of poor planetary health is the impact on human health. Environmental factors such as air and water pollution, exposure to harmful chemicals, and climate change–related events can have serious implications for human well-being. For example, air pollution has been linked to respiratory diseases such as asthma and chronic obstructive pulmonary disease, as well as cardiovascular issues and even premature death. Contaminated water sources can lead to a host of waterborne diseases, while exposure to toxic chemicals can result in a range of health problems, including cancer, neurological disorders, and reproductive issues.

Climate change, which is a key driver of planetary health concerns, has numerous consequences for human populations. Rising global temperatures contribute to more frequent and more severe heatwaves, which can be particularly dangerous for vulnerable populations such as the elderly and those with pre-existing health conditions. Changes in climate patterns can also lead to food and water insecurity, as shifting precipitation patterns and increased frequency of extreme weather events can disrupt agricultural systems and water supplies.

In addition to the direct impact on human health, poor planetary health can also have profound social and economic consequences. Environmental degradation can exacerbate social inequalities, as marginalised communities are often disproportionately affected by pollution and climate-related disasters. Displacement due to environmental factors such as droughts or floods can lead to conflict and instability, further undermining social cohesion and economic development.

From an economic perspective, the consequences of poor planetary health are manifold. The degradation of natural resources and ecosystems can disrupt supply chains, leading to food shortages, reduced agricultural productivity, and increased competition for essential resources. The cost of responding to environmental disasters and mitigating the effects of climate change can be staggering, straining national budgets and diverting resources away from other critical areas such as health care and education.

Furthermore, the loss of biodiversity and degradation of ecosystems can have cascading effects on the functioning of our planet. Ecosystem services such as pollination, water purification, and carbon sequestration are essential for human well-being, and their decline can have far-reaching consequences for global ecosystems and economies (The Asia Foundation, 2021).

In conclusion, the consequences of poor planetary health are vast and wide-ranging, impacting human health, social structures, economies, and ecosystems. By recognising the interconnectedness of environmental sustainability and human well-being, we can work towards creating a more resilient and sustainable future for all. It is imperative that we take action to address the root causes of environmental degradation and prioritise the health of our planet for the well-being of current and future generations.

1.8 Social Security and Planetary Health

Social security and planetary health are two critical aspects of human well-being that are deeply interconnected. Social security encompasses a range of policies and programs designed to provide economic support and assistance to individuals and communities in times of need, while planetary health focuses on the health of the environment and its impact on human health. Understanding the relationship between these two concepts is crucial for creating a sustainable and resilient future for all.

One key area where social security and planetary health intersect is in the context of climate change and environmental degradation. Climate change is a global phenomenon that poses significant risks to human populations, ecosystems, and economies (Goel et al., 2020). Rising global temperatures, more frequent and severe natural disasters, and shifts in precipitation patterns all have implications for food security, water availability, and human health. Social security programs play a vital role in helping communities adapt to and recover from the impacts of climate change, providing essential support to those most affected by environmental disasters and disruptions.

For example, in the aftermath of a natural disaster such as a hurricane or wildfire, social security programs such as emergency relief funds, food assistance programs, and temporary housing assistance can help affected individuals and communities rebuild their lives and regain their footing. These programs not only provide immediate relief to those in need but also contribute to long-term recovery and resilience by addressing underlying vulnerabilities and promoting sustainable practices.

Furthermore, the concept of social security is closely tied to issues of environmental justice and equity. Marginalised communities, including low-income populations, minorities, and Indigenous peoples, are often disproportionately affected by environmental hazards and pollution. These communities may lack access to clean air and water, face higher rates of exposure to toxic chemicals, and be more vulnerable to the health impacts of climate change. Social security programs must be designed and implemented in a way that addresses these disparities and ensures that all individuals have equal access to essential services and support.

In addition to the role of social security in addressing the impacts of environmental degradation, planetary health considerations are also increasingly relevant in the design and implementation of social security programs. For example, promoting sustainable agriculture practices, investing in renewable energy sources, and improving public transportation systems can all contribute to a healthier planet and a more resilient society. By integrating planetary health principles into social security policies, we can create more effective and sustainable solutions to the challenges we face.

Moreover, the concept of social security extends beyond traditional welfare programs to encompass broader issues of social well-being and economic security. In a world facing growing environmental challenges such as climate change, biodiversity loss, and water scarcity, social security programs must adapt to address these new risks and vulnerabilities. This may involve expanding access to health care services, strengthening social safety nets, and promoting sustainable economic development practices that prioritise the well-being of people and the planet.

In conclusion, social security and planetary health are intricately linked concepts that are essential for creating a more equitable, sustainable, and resilient future. By recognising the interconnections between human well-being, environmental sustainability, and social equity, we can develop more effective policies and programs that address the complex challenges of the 21st century. It is imperative that we prioritise the health of both people and the planet in our decision-making processes and work towards a more just and sustainable society for all.

1.9 Conclusion

In conclusion the idea of health provides an insightful understanding of how closely linked the well-being of our planet is to the health of its inhabitants. This chapter recognises that environmental factors affecting our planet—such as air quality, climate change, biodiversity loss and disruptions, to ecosystems—are intricately connected to human health.

The COVID-19 pandemic has made it clear that there is a need to prioritise the health of both individuals and the planet. It has shown how important it is to protect biodiversity and ecosystems to prevent the spread of diseases from animals to humans. Governments and international organisations play a role in promoting planetary health by implementing comprehensive policies and governance structures as seen in initiatives like the Paris Agreement and the United Nations Sustainable Development Goals.

Looking ahead, there is an opportunity after the pandemic to adopt a more sustainable and fair approach to health care. By focusing on health, we can not only improve public health outcomes and be better prepared for future pandemics but also encourage preventive measures, healthier lifestyles, and sustainable practices.

By recognising and taking action on the interconnectedness between health and environmental health we can pave the way for a brighter future that is sustainable. Planetary health provides a roadmap, towards achieving well-being, where individual well-being goes hand in hand with the well-being of the planet. This ensures a more resilient and fairer world for generations to come.

Bibliography

Centers for Disease Control and Prevention. (2022). *Similarities and differences between Flu and COVID-19*. Retrieved March 7, 2022, from https://www.cdc.gov/flu/symptoms/flu-vs-covid19.htm

Drake, J. (2021, April 22). What is planetary health? *Forbes*. Retrieved July 19, 2023, from https://www.forbes.com/sites/johndrake/2021/04/22/what-is-planetary-health/?sh=4e0bc07d2998

Goel, K., Arora, A., Rehman, T., Angchuk, P., Samphel, R., Kiran, T., Padhi, B. K.., Rajagopal, V., & Thakur, J. S. (2020). The successful containment of COVID-19 outbreak in Union Territory of Ladakh, India, 2020. *Journal of Family Medicine and Primary Care*, *9*(11), 5574. https://doi.org/10.4103/jfmpc.jfmpc_1413_20

Haines et al., (2015). Nurturing children's healthy eating: Position statement. Appetite, 137, 124–133. https://doi.org/10.1016/j.appet.2019.02.007.

Mahmood, J. (2023, April 22). A 'whole of nation' effort. *The Star*. Retrieved July 26, 2023, from https://www.thestar.com.my/news/environment/2023/04/22/a-whole-of-nation-effort

Mahmood, J., & Guinto, R. R. (2022, February 8). Indonesia: Why planetary health should be on the menu for the G20 chair. *Think Global Health*. Retrieved July 26, 2023, from https://www.thinkglobalhealth.org/article/indonesia-why-planetary-health-should-be-menu-g20-chair

Di Marco, M., Harwood, T. D., Hoskins, A. J., Ware, C., Hill, S. L. L., & Ferrier, S. (2019). Projecting impacts of global climate and land-use scenarios on plant biodiversity using compositional-turnover modelling. *Global Change Biology*, *25*, 2763–2778.

Intergovernmental Panel on Climate Change-IPCC (2018). V. Masson, et al. Cambridge University Press. https://doi.org/10.1017/9781009157940

Iyer, L. R. (2021). A cross-cultural dialogue to save the planet: Realizing Sustainable Development Goals 2030. *Journal of Dharma*, *46*(2), 1–20.

Mirza, A., & Rauhala, E. (2021). Here's just how unequal the global coronavirus vaccine rollout has been. *Washington Post*. Retrieved March 7, 2022, from https://www.washingtonpost.com/world/interactive/2021/coronavirus-vaccine-inequality-global/

Mukherjee, S. (2021). Why does the pandemic seem to be hitting some countries harder than others? *The New Yorker*. Retrieved March 15, 2022, from https://www.newyorker.com/magazine/2021/03/01/why-does-the-pandemic-seem-to-be-hitting-some-countries-harder-than-others

Myers, S. S. (2017). Planetary health: Protecting human health on a rapidly changing planet. *The Lancet*, *390*(10114), 2860–2868.

Nagarik Network. (2020). Nepal-China Rasuwagadhi border point to be sealed for 15 days from Wednesday. Retrieved March 7, 2022, from https://myrepublica.nagariknetwork.com/news/85919/

Neuman, S. (2021). COVID-19 reaches mount Everest as Nepal struggles with record infections. *National Public Radio (NPR)*. Retrieved November 24, 2021, from https://www.npr.org/sections/coronavirus-live-updates/2021/05/05/993837355/covid-19-reaches-mount-everest-as-nepal-struggles-with-record-infections

Oehler, R., & Vega, V. (2021). Conquering COVID: How global vaccine inequality risks prolonging the pandemic. *Open Forum Infectious Diseases*, *8*(10). https://doi.org/10.1093/ofid/ofab443

Pun, S., Mandal, S., Bhandari, L., Jha, S., Rajbhandari, S., Mishra, A. K., Sharma Chalise, B., & Shah, R. (2020). Understanding COVID-19 in Nepal. *Journal of Nepal Health Research Council*, *18*(1), 126–127. https://doi.org/10.33314/jnhrc.v18i1.2629

Ranjit, S., Sigdel, S., Ozaki, A., Kotera, Y., Bhandari, D., Regmi, P., & Rabaan, A. (2020). Impact of COVID-19 on tourism in Nepal. *Journal of Travel Medicine*, *27*(6). Retrieved November 25, 2021, from https://academic.oup.com/jtm/article/27/6/taaa105/5868304.

Reuters. (2021). COVID-19 tracker: Bhutan. Retrieved November 24, 2021, from https://graphics.reuters.com/world-coronavirus-tracker-and-maps/countries-and-territories/bhutan/.

Royal Government of Bhutan. (2022). *Vaccines for Bhutan*. Retrieved from https://www.gov.bt/covid19/13-07-21-Press-Release-Vac/

Schiffling, S., & Phelan, C. (2021). What the world can learn from Bhutan's rapid COVID vaccine rollout. *The Conversation*. Retrieved from https://theconversation.com/what-the-world-can-learn-from-bhutans-rapid-covid-vaccine-rollout-168341

Schoff, A., Joshi, K., Adhikari, P., & Pant, G. (2020). The effect of the COVID-19 pandemic on mountain communities of the Indian Himalaya. *Mountain Sentinels*. Retrieved November 24, 2021, from https://mountainsentinels.org/the-effect-of-the-covid-19-pandemic-on-mountain-communities-of-the-indian-himalaya/

Shrestha, S. (2021). Nepal says its Covid response is under control – everyone can see it's not true. *The Guardian*. Retrieved November 24, 2021, from https://www.theguardian.com/global-development/commentisfree/2021/may/11/nepal-says-its-covid-response-is-under-control-everyone-can-see-its-not-true

Syailendrawati, R., Chan, A., Leach-Kemon, K., & Mokdad, A. (2022). *What happens when zero-COVID countries lift restrictions: How Singapore, Australia, Vietnam, and others are transitioning*. Council on Foreign Relation. Retrieved from https://www.thinkglobalhealth.org/article/what-happens-when-zero-covid-countries-lift-restrictions

Tamang, S., & Dorji, T. (2021). Challenges and response to the second major local outbreak of COVID-19 in Bhutan. *Asia Pacific Journal of Public Health*, *33*(8), 953–955. Retrieved November 25, 2021, from https://pubmed.ncbi.nlm.nih.gov/33829879/

The Asia Foundation. (2021). *The impact of the covid-19 pandemic on employment in middle-order cities of Nepal a Rapid Assessment.* The Asia Foundation. Retrieved from https://asiafoundation.org/wp-content/uploads/2021/04/Impact-of-the-Covid-19-Pandemic-on-Employment-in-Middle-order-Cities-of-Nepal.pdf

United Nations. (2015). Transforming our world: The 2030 Agenda for Sustainable Development. UN General Assembly.

Watts, N., Adger, W. N., Agnolucci, P., Blackstock, J., Byass, P., Cai, W., Chaytor, S., Colbourn, T., Collins, M., Cooper, A., Cox, P. M., Depledge, J., Drummond, P., Ekins, P., Galaz, V., Grace, D., Graham, H., Grubb, M., Haines, A., … Costello, A. (2015). Health and climate change: Policy responses to protect public health. *The Lancet, 386*(10006), 1861–1914.

Whitmee, S., Haines, A., Beyrer, C., Boltz, F., Capon, A. G., de Souza Dias, B. F., Ezeh, A., Frumkin, H., Gong, P., Head, P., Horton, R., Mace, G. M., Marten, R., Myers, S. S., Nishtar, S., Osofsky, S. A., Pattanayak, S. K., Pongsiri, M. J., Romanelli, C., … Yach, D. (2015). Safeguarding human health in the Anthropocene epoch: Report of the Rockefeller Foundation–Lancet Commission on planetary health. *The Lancet, 386*(10007), 1973–2028.

Wilcox, B. A., et al. (2019). Disease transmission in the Anthropocene: Zoonotic emergence and the role of global travel and trade. *Trends in Parasitology, 35*(7), 607–616.

Willetts, E., & de Paula, N. (2021). International Institute for Sustainable Development. *Still Only One Earth.* Retrieved July 19, 2023, from https://www.iisd.org/system/files/2021-03/still-one-earth-health.pdf

Withers, M., Cousineau, M., Hairi, N. N., Rampal, S., & Wipfl, H. (2020). The Kuala Lumpur statement on planetary health from the Association of Pacific Rim Universities Global Health Program. *ASM Science Journal, 13*(5), 3–6.

World Health Organisation. (2022). *Nepal: WHO coronavirus disease (COVID-19) dashboard with vaccination data.* Retrieved March 7, 2022, from https://covid19.who.int/region/searo/country/np

Zinsstag, J., Schelling, E., Waltner-Toews, D., & Tanner, M. (2011). From "one medicine" to "one health" and systemic approaches to health and well-being. *Journal of Preventive Veterinary Medicine, 101*(3-4):148–156.

2

PLANETARY HEALTH

A Revised View on Healthy Living

Muhd Nabhan Mizan

2.1 Introduction

The world has undergone numerous global transformations, yet few compare to the profound modernisation ushered in by the Industrial Revolution of the 19th century. Enthralled by the promise of a new era driven by globalised market systems, nations swiftly embraced industrialisation, triggering widespread carbon emissions through large-scale production processes. Initially a niche concern among scientists studying environmental changes and natural disasters, the emphasis on healthy, sustainable living has since become a mainstream priority. It now occupies a central position in multi-level discussions, from classrooms and youth initiatives to deliberations among world leaders (Özdemir, 2019).

Recognising the pervasive impacts of climate change and the necessity of international collaboration, United Nations-led initiatives have resulted in the adoption of landmark frameworks such as the Sustainable Development Goals (SDGs) and the 2015 Paris Agreement—the first legally binding international accord under the United Nations Framework Convention on Climate Change (UNFCCC) to address climate change comprehensively. These agreements serve as critical guidelines for promoting sustainable practices, reshaping consumer behaviour, and stimulating market growth. More recently, refined strategies such as the Environmental, Social, and Governance (ESG) framework, widely adopted by multinational corporations, have emerged. Simultaneously, alternative measures of human progress, such as the Human Development Index (HDI), have shifted the focus from GDP growth alone to prioritise equity and human well-being. These approaches pave the way towards achieving the Paris Agreement's target of limiting global temperature rise to well below two degrees Celsius.

DOI: 10.4324/9781003569084-3

Regrettably, recent findings from the United Nations Framework Convention on Climate Change (UNFCC) indicate that, based on ongoing endeavours, there is a projected likelihood of surpassing the advised temperature increase of one degree by the Intergovernmental Panel on Climate Change (IPCC) by the conclusion of the present century (Saier, 2022). Despite ongoing efforts, more than the current reduction in initial carbon dioxide (CO_2) emissions is needed to ensure the long-term viability of the environment (Saier, 2022). Crawley et al. (2021) performed research that revealed that, so far, drivers of sustainability have erroneously conflated societal ideas with problem salience. It is often held that the recognition of the adverse effects of climate change on human existence by a majority of individuals should therefore result in a prevailing public sentiment favouring measures to address climate change (Crawley et al., 2021). Rather, it is subject to the effect of issue salience and how the public perceives and evaluates it in comparison to other matters. A significant proportion of individuals, particularly in economically disadvantaged countries, choose immediate survival above long-term intangible advantages. This inclination is reflected in their voting patterns concerning economic and political proposals.

One of the greatest challenges facing global action on climate change is the issue of localised implementation. Several factors contribute to this, including insufficient data, limited expertise, and inadequate budgets—issues that collectively fall under the umbrella term 'saliency'. Moreover, the adoption of sustainable practices is deeply intertwined with political priorities, often competing with short-term goals deemed more pressing by society. As a result, governments are frequently pressured to prioritise policies aimed at enhancing immediate personal wealth, thereby compromising long-term 'greater' objectives. This prioritisation trickles down to influence local rules, regulations, and budgets, diverting resources that could otherwise support sustainability initiatives. The financial burden of sustainable living further complicates its adoption, particularly in poorer nations that are disproportionately vulnerable to climate change and ill-equipped to bear its costs (Crawley et al., 2021). International discussions are often stalled in a blame game over responsibility for climate action, exacerbating the challenge and fostering growing pessimism among the youth regarding a sustainable future. However, the rise in natural disasters, such as the Hawaii wildfires and flooding in Pakistan, should not deter efforts to combat climate change. Every reduction in global temperature, even by a fraction of a degree, delays the tipping point of no return, extending the viability of Earth and humanity's existence.

In response to growing concerns about the intersection of environmental and human health, the concept of planetary health was introduced in 2015. The UK-based medical journal *The Lancet* launched a commission in collaboration with the Rockefeller Foundation to address this emerging field, culminating in the report *Safeguarding Human Health in the Anthropocene Period* (Planetary Health Alliance, 2015). This report underscores how humanity has significantly benefited from alterations to the Earth's natural systems, such as increased life expectancies and poverty reduction (Planetary Health Alliance, 2015). However, it also warns that these economic and developmental gains have come at the expense of future generations' health, leaving us to confront their dire consequences (Planetary Health Alliance, 2023). Professor Andy Haines, a pioneer of Planetary Health, emphasised in an interview with *The Lancet* that the Planetary Health Alliance provides a coherent conceptual framework. This framework aims to balance the promotion of human health with the necessity of living within the Earth's environmental boundaries, advocating for sustainable practices that protect both current and future generations

A key strength of planetary health is that it is not a completely new field of study. Rather than calling for entirely new initiatives, it offers a perspective that encourages individuals and organisations across various sectors to consider the broader, interconnected picture. Instead of requiring a complete overhaul of existing systems, it builds upon them, fostering an understanding of their interdependencies. This approach helps bridge the gap between experts and end-users in diverse fields, facilitating collaboration and shared understanding. However, this integrative perspective introduces new challenges, such as achieving consensus among a wide array of stakeholders. Planetary health must compete for attention alongside numerous other pressing issues faced by these stakeholders, raising questions about saliency and priority-setting. It acknowledges the complexities of implementing effective climate action policies at both local and international levels, recognising the obstacles inherent in translating global goals into actionable and context-specific measures.

2.2   Why Planetary Health?

As discussed above, the focus on combating climate change has gained unprecedented prominence, with green efforts taking centre stage more than ever before. This raises the question of why the term 'planetary health' has emerged and why it warrants attention. For a long time, public health has been viewed through a traditional, siloed lens, often perceived as the exclusive domain of doctors, scientists, and physicists (Myers, 2017, pp. 2860–2868). Nevertheless, adopting a fragmented perspective when addressing public health poses a significant risk to the efficacy of public health initiatives, as it hampers inclusion and inhibits the interchange of ideas among experts from other disciplines. Public health problems often go unnoticed or disregarded in policy implementation, despite studies urging prompt action by policymakers. Throughout the succession of environmental summits convened throughout the years, a recurring theme emerged, namely the insufficiency of our actions and the delayed implementation of promised initiatives.

The subject of issue salience is brought up in this context. There is a significant disparity between climate change belief and issue salience among the general public. In a survey conducted by Crawley et al. (2019), despite an overwhelming majority of respondents believing that climate change is occurring and that the government must take appropriate action, only 17% rank it among the top three issues. When such a figure is exhibited by climate action leaders like the United Kingdom, it is concerning for nations with less developed and stable economic, political, and social dynamics. It is also essential to recognise that issue salience varies based on localised emergency threats (Spisak et al., 2022). During the Covid-19 pandemic, the salience of climate change decreased, in contrast to when wildfires and droughts received pervasive media coverage (Spisak et al., 2022). Based on research by the World Economic Forum, Stantcheva (2024) describes that societies tend to prioritise short-term benefits over long-term environmental impacts as their consequences are not immediately apparent. This ephemeral character of issue salience is a reflection on how personal survival dominates decision making (Stantcheva, 2024). Green policies have faced and still face a tug of war with more immediate and popular concerns, such as economic growth, political agendas, and social priorities (Bromley-Trujillo & Poe, 2018).

Planetary Health addresses this challenge by advocating a shift in our perception of the Earth's ecosystems and their intrinsic value. This emerging concept emphasises that climate action must transcend specialised fields such as health and medicine, integrating sustainability into decision-making processes across all sectors. The Planetary Health Commission urges a holistic approach, encouraging individuals and organisations to consider their impact on the environment before prioritising personal or institutional gains. Echoing the words of activist Wendell Berry, "[W]hat is good for the Earth will be good for us, not the other way around" (Horton & Lo, 2015, pp. 1921–1922).

Over the past decades, academic literature has extensively documented the profound impact of human activity on the planet, from the Industrial Revolution's rapid mechanisation of daily life to globalisation's reshaping of the distribution of goods and services worldwide. Environmentalists have consistently emphasised the detrimental effects of human actions, particularly the overexploitation of the Earth's finite resources. This unsustainable global ecological footprint must not continue, as it perpetuates harmful biophysical changes that prioritise short-term gains over the long-term well-being of future generations, echoing the issue of saliency previously discussed (Myers, 2017, pp. 2860–2868). This epoch of significant human influence, referred to as the Anthropocene, has historically been addressed through various environmental frameworks. These approaches often operate under the assumption that humans alone are the primary drivers of environmental change—a perspective that is both reductive and inadequate (Myers, 2017, pp. 2860–2868; Özdemir, 2019). The Earth's ecosystem is far more complex, consisting of the dynamic interaction of countless interconnected subsystems. For example, while the construction of hydroelectric dams is often criticised for deforestation-related soil erosion and water pollution, a planetary health perspective also considers the disruption of fishing income upon degradation of marine ecosystems, shaping future economic patterns.

Consider the case of biofuel production. The development of renewable energy is often regarded as an innovative method for fuel production, resulting in a corresponding decrease in the utilisation of fossil fuels and the associated environmental consequences. Nevertheless, its advocates have overlooked the economic drawbacks of biofuel. Extensive research has shown that alterations in land utilisation and feedstock selection have resulted in a rise in greenhouse gas (GHG) emissions and a surge in food costs (US EPA, 2014). Moreover, lax regulatory practices have exacerbated the negative impact of green policies on the environment, as shown by the case of the tree planting subsidy scheme in Chile. The present investigation examined the implications of promoting tree-planting initiatives aimed at establishing new forests, revealing a consequential reduction in the area of native forests and a subsequent decline in biodiversity (Heilmayr et al., 2020). To address the discrepancies in the efficacy of climate action, it is imperative to recognise that prior approaches to environmental well-being, predicated on the notion that human beings are the exclusive catalysts of the Earth's systems, represent an inadequate and simplistic understanding of the interconnected dynamics of our surroundings (Özdemir, 2019). The Earth's ecosystem is comprised of the simultaneous interplay of several ecosystems. The construction of hydroelectric dams warrants consideration. The construction of a large-scale infrastructure project might be seen as potentially resulting in water and soil contamination as a consequence of deforestation, hence posing a future risk of landslides and adverse impacts on human well-being. Nevertheless, a scholar specialising in planetary health would duly recognise and take into account the intricate relationship between marine life habitats and the alteration in soil nutrient composition resulting from the decline in tree root anchorage capacity.

The principle of planetary health advocates for the involvement of specialists from various academic disciplines in promoting the well-being of the Earth's ecosystems, encompassing all forms of life. It emphasises the human responsibility to act as stewards of these ecosystems, ensuring their health and vitality. This notion is exemplified by the real-life case study of groundwater salinity in Bangladesh, as discussed by Ozdemir (2019) and Myers (2017, pp. 2860–2868). The study primarily aimed to assess the effects of elevated salt content in groundwater resulting from sea level rise, severe storms, and the construction of dams upstream (Khan et al., 2008). The study conducted by Khan et al. (2008) showed a clear correlation between the saline levels of groundwater in coastal regions of Bangladesh and the occurrence of pre-eclampsia, gestational hypertension in pregnant women, and a general rise in high blood pressure. The field of planetary health recognises the importance of complicated natural processes to comprehend their potential bad repercussions, even if they are distant, particularly concerning public health.

Given the prevailing state of our environmental, economic, and political systems, it is evident that our society is poised to confront significant repercussions stemming from climate change. These implications have been exacerbated by the sluggish pace of action and the inadequacy of tactics used thus far in addressing climate-related challenges. For many decades leading up to the present, it can be argued that our society has mostly fostered conditions that disproportionately favour a select group of affluent people (Horton et al., 2014, p. 847). The field of planetary health is concerned with addressing environmental challenges and advocating for equitable climate action, aiming to ensure that all individuals have equal access to a healthy planetary ecosystem. Within this particular movement, there is a deliberate focus on addressing matters of justice and equality. This emphasis is driven by the recognition of the need to diminish disparities in vulnerability that exist throughout various cultures (Myers, 2017, pp. 2860–2868). While the primary underlying elements contributing to environmental catastrophes are often attributed to insufficient or delayed climate action, it is essential to acknowledge that in the immediate term, the survival and resilience of civilisation are influenced by several variables, including governance, wealth, technology improvements, and individual behaviour.

Although the call for a shared responsibility against global warming is widely supported, different societies have not contributed equally to the current pollution levels, with developing countries suffering the most from the past pollution of current economic powerhouses (Guzmán et al., 2021). For example, while clean energy initiatives, such as dam construction, may appear beneficial to urban populations relying on hydroelectric power, they often exacerbate health risks for vulnerable communities, such as increased exposure to schistosomiasis. Planetary Health emphasises the importance of conducting health impact assessments that account for the diverse effects across different societies and explicitly address issues of equity. Therefore, the Commission calls for us to look beyond the demands and needs of our current societies and expand the realm of public health to include how we steward the earth's natural ecosystems. Achieving such a holistic approach requires interdisciplinary collaboration among researchers, public health practitioners, and policymakers. Partnerships that transcend traditional public health boundaries are essential (Myers, 2017, pp. 2860–2868). Furthermore, the reorganisation of public health education is necessary to foster interdepartmental cooperation at all levels of training (Guzmán et al., 2021; Myers, 2017, pp. 2860–2868). Bias in academic publications must also be minimised through the provision of adequate cross-disciplinary funding, ensuring that global health challenges are addressed comprehensively and without the constraints of siloed perspectives (Myers, 2017, pp. 2860–2868).

The current state of affairs does not align with a scenario in which all functional systems exist in isolation from one another (Pongsiri et al., 2017). The examination of public health necessitates the inclusion of political factors, much like the interconnectedness seen with social justice (Pongsiri et al., 2017). The Commission posits that by redefining our methods of observation and treatment of the earth's ecosystems, we might enhance our comprehension and appreciation of them, leading to the establishment of a more profound relationship with the natural world. The resolution of the longstanding disconnection among specialists from many disciplines has the potential to enhance decision-making processes and facilitate the implementation of policies with more efficacy across all domains.

2.3 Understanding the Planetary Health Framework in Sectors

The successful implementation of planetary health requires an extensive understanding of its underlying foundation. The planetary health paradigm takes a systems approach that supports the concept that health is the interplay between natural and social systems (Pongsiri et al., 2017). This perspective aligns with the significant responsibility that humankind has as the agent of influence over global biological systems. The adoption of a systems-based approach may be accomplished by implementing the practice of stewarding biological systems. This approach has the potential to not only mitigate our excessive exploitative consumer behaviours but also transform ecosystems into more robust and environmentally sustainable systems (Pongsiri et al., 2017). The technique discussed in this study focuses on three primary areas, with the first being the examination of system complexity (Pongsiri et al., 2017). The examination of system complexity entails the evaluation and ongoing reevaluation of climate change strategies over extended temporal intervals. These assessments must factor in the short-term and long-term consequences and the possible adverse effects on all sentient beings, incorporating the spirit of equity and justice. By examining sudden and drastic changes in ecosystems, it becomes possible to prevent permanent harm to both natural systems and human well-being. It is well-recognised that the field of environmental science is experiencing significant growth and will likely continue to grow in the future. The accessibility of newly enhanced and cost-effective green technologies will require our readiness to integrate these advancements when required.

An additional factor that needs consideration is the recognition of the significant influence exerted by humans in shaping our understanding of socioecological systems. The significance of framing information is of great importance as it has a major influence on technical progress, social attitudes towards climate change, and therefore the potential of subsequent climate action (Pongsiri et al., 2017). The construction of this body of knowledge is evident in both official and informal educational settings, various media outlets, policy development processes, and, notably, scholarly writing. We cannot see that our present is exclusive to the past and future. In reality, the present conditions of living are the consequences of past conditions of living. It is essential to ensure the incorporation of this ethos at all stages of decision-making across diverse industries. In order to do this, it would be necessary to include a diversified range of professionals from many sectors, including social scientists, medical practitioners, civil society representatives, and policymakers (Pongsiri et al., 2017). Climate action plans would be better developed as a result, producing a common knowledge of the systems underpinning decision-making and governance processes that could genuinely drive changes at the implementation level.

Finally, the systems approach necessitates the consideration of upstream drivers that contribute to adverse environmental effects. According to Pongsiri et al. (2017), the field of planetary health argues that existing strategies for addressing climate change have been limited in their focus on the immediate causes of pollution, thereby neglecting the broader range of elements that contribute to these activities. In order to effectively tackle the problem of illicit logging in developing nations, it is imperative to go beyond the mere incarceration of those engaged in this activity. Instead, it is crucial to delve into the underlying factors that drive the demand for illegal logging and hinder the inclination of these individuals to pursue legitimate employment prospects. This paradigm shift fundamentally reimagines human interactions with the planet's resources and how climate actions themselves are designed, enhancing their efficacy.

Evidently, implementing planetary health via the systems approach would require changes in the way we assess system complexity, upholding the massive responsibility that humanity has as stewards of those complex systems, and delving deeper into the possible upstream drivers of planetary health. To take a systemic approach, it is necessary to alter the dynamics of the system and use various tools related to planetary health. These tools may include the integration of spatially explicit land-use models and ecosystem services models (Pongsiri et al., 2017). By adopting this approach, the study of climate action will facilitate more effective planning, ascertain mutually beneficial solutions that cater to diverse sectors, and ultimately assist in optimising policy interventions throughout the implementation phase. Thus far, we have engaged in a discourse pertaining to the conceptualisation and implementation of the systems approach in the context of planetary health, as well as providing a comprehensive synopsis of the prospective advantages associated with its adoption. This approach must now be spilt over and influence the framework of different sectors (i.e., education, medicine, economy, and governance) to place planetary health at the centre of their decision-making process. The subsequent subsections will elucidate the functioning of planetary-health-integrated frameworks within the domains of education and governance. It is hoped that these guidelines will serve as a versatile framework for our adoption of them while also providing insights into the possible advantages and obstacles associated with their implementation.

2.3.1 Education

Education is one of the most essential areas in which planetary health should be incorporated. Education has a crucial and indispensable role in imparting knowledge and understanding of planetary health concepts to aspiring future leaders, hence shaping our attitude towards climate action. If we were to exclude it from education, we may shape a generation that fails to factor in the importance of taking a systems approach to planetary health and the continuation of ineffective policies. Consequently, within this particular segment of the article, I want to emphasise the planetary health education framework put forward by the elected task force of the Planetary Health Alliance, as provided by Guzmán et al. (2021). The proposed framework promotes the systematic incorporation of planetary health into various academic disciplines and educational levels. It emphasises the importance of structured integration while also allowing for adaptable implementation at the local level, in alignment with the suggested educational domains. Consequently, the implementation of planetary health education would enable present-day learners to acquire the essential information and attitude required to initiate transdisciplinary efforts aimed at addressing the declining state of planetary health. The framework has five domains that interact with each other and together serve as a roadmap for education, equipping young individuals with an appreciation for the interdependent nature of these domains (Guzmán et al., 2021).

First of all, the interconnection within nature. The paradigm emphasises the importance of education in cultivating a profound and meaningful relationship with the natural world, positioning it as a central aspect within the five domains. The aforementioned approach stresses the notion that education is not just characterised by a unidirectional transmission of information but rather contains elements of affect and interpersonal connections within the educational context (Guzmán et al., 2021). To effectively tackle the problem of climate change, it is imperative to first examine the fundamental nature of our connection with the Earth. Amidst the routines of our daily lives and our pursuit of enhanced living conditions, it is sometimes overlooked that our planet offers essential resources such as forests, rivers, and seas, which are vital for human sustenance. This field promotes the idea of educators seeking inspiration from the ideals upheld by non-capitalist Indigenous cultures, which emphasise profound ties with the natural world (Guzmán et al., 2021). The knowledge and spiritual connections within these communities have the potential to enhance planetary health education by using an educational method that resonates more deeply with learners, fostering a genuine feeling of affection for the planet as its fundamental basis. As a result, there may be an increased appreciation for climate action.

Education on planetary health cannot be conducted without emphasising the roles humans have played throughout time in shaping the current world—be it for the better or worse (Guzmán et al., 2021). Hence, it is of utmost significance that education integrates the realms of the Anthropocene and health. While a significant proportion of the populace acknowledges the occurrence of climate change and recognises the substantial human influence on it, public confidence in the institutions and experts engaged in climate research exhibits considerable polarisation. Tranter et al. (2023) provide empirical support for the proposition that Australians exhibit scepticism about the Intergovernmental Panel on Climate Change (IPCC) and see possible individual gains for scientists in the context of climate research. The erosion of public confidence has adverse implications for public attitudes and actions in climate mitigation endeavours (Tranter et al., 2023). Support for mitigation policies is also negated by the growing negative perception of climate pressure groups such as Just Stop Oil and efforts by major production companies to control the public narrative for fossil fuels. The lobbying practices of major oil corporations and their deliberate efforts to redirect public attention away from climate action to maintain a consistent demand for non-renewable energy sources are explored in a report conducted by BBC Channel 4 (Thompson, 2021). Consequently, the experience of helplessness arises, prompting individuals to persist in their prevailing consuming behaviours, thus diminishing the efficacy of environmental education. This paradigm prioritises the comprehension of the interconnections between human influences on Earth's natural systems and health consequences. It further builds upon the knowledge of the fundamental elements that amplify or mitigate these effects. By acquiring this comprehension, learners will develop a heightened level of consciousness, enabling them to make decisions that take into account the anthropogenic effects on the surrounding systems.

Now that learners have an understanding of how humans have and still influence the natural systems occurring around us, they must enhance that knowledge by understanding how these different systems interact with one another. With this, planetary health demands that education embed systems thinking and complexity in their teachings (Guzmán et al., 2021). In the subsection on the systems approach, we outline how it works and how we may model it for use in different sectoral frameworks. This information must now be conveyed to learners of planetary health so that they can characterise the different linkages between environmental changes and human health at different geospatial and temporal scales (Guzmán et al., 2021). This form of learning would require them to have a grasp of complex adaptive systems such as circular causal relationships, emerging characteristics, and self-organisation (Guzmán et al., 2021). Learners must also be equipped with the self-awareness of having biases in decision-making and the necessary skills to overcome them. With this, the values of justice and equity must also be embedded in education so that learners are aware of how the current working systems only benefit a small group of rich people (Guzmán et al., 2021).

To achieve equity and justice, systemic disparities must be eliminated so that no society faces disproportionate health and environmental burdens due to climate change. The educational process must nurture an adequate understanding of extant structural inequities and how historical political, economic, and social injustices have influenced contemporary society and environmental impacts (Guzmán et al., 2021). Future planetary health practitioners will be prepared to implement structural changes in institutions that promote and perpetuate inequities and shape planetary living conditions if they are inculcated with the values of equity and justice (Guzmán et al., 2021). Integration of movement-building and systems-change strategies into education is the final step. (Guzmán et al., 2021) Change does not occur on its own and requires adequate skills in movement development. These actions necessitate an understanding of inclusive relationships, deliberate strategies, effective communication, and transformative partnerships so that future professionals can potentially create effective movements to support system change (Guzmán et al., 2021).

According to research conducted by the International Monetary Fund (IMF) and authored by Dabla-Norris et al. (2023), there exists a notable disparity between public perception and the level of endorsement for climate policy pertaining to mitigation efforts. A considerable segment of the populace, particularly in developing nations, recognises the significance of prompt mitigation measures and their present affliction due to climate change (Dabla-Norris et al., 2023). Nevertheless, there is a discernible discrepancy in the formulation of these policies, their communication strategies to the public, and the explicit methods used for their implementation (Dabla-Norris et al., 2023). The incorporation of a planetary health perspective in the field of education would contribute to this goal by fostering a thorough understanding of the many systems and processes involved in mitigation efforts, as well as the historical repercussions that have shaped the present environmental conditions. Overall, this pedagogical framework for planetary health allows institutions, educators, and students to integrate values that are both structural and adaptable. These modifications would enable institutions to adapt this guiding framework to their level of expertise and capacity, resulting in more locally relevant instructional materials. The delivery of education will include trans-disciplinary context-based instruction and will prepare platforms for youth to engage in transformative partnerships. As a result, we will be able to cultivate a generation of learners that abandons the conventional, compartmentalised approach to education and moves towards a prospering environment for all.

2.3.2   Governance

The significance of planetary health education is exemplified by its role in preparing future leaders of environmental change with knowledge tied to the reality of inequity and injustice, as well as with change-appropriate skills. However, such a change cannot be implemented unless governance is adapted to accommodate planetary health. Governance encompasses issues on management, how we facilitate the process of adopting planetary health frameworks, and resource capacity. This reflects the planetary health belief that health transcends the human body and is essentially everywhere (Gabrys, 2020). Planetary health interacts and integrates with, among other factors, the environment, urban development, education, transportation policies, and national politics (Gabrys, 2020). It must be emphasised that achieving planetary health does not merely entail rebranding global or environmental health as planetary health; rather, it requires a governance approach to environmental issues that takes into account aspects of justice and local management capacities (Gabrys, 2020). We have reached a point in environmental management where reducing our ecological imprints is no longer sufficient, and we must inculcate a planetary health perspective at all levels of government. This is the reason why planetary health governance goes beyond the identification of direct causes of degrading environments and also investigates drivers of human cooperation and the capacities to act on them (Horton & Lo, 2015, pp. 1921–1922). The planetary health governance framework is designed to address three main issues: the transition from public to planetary health, the relationship between science and politics, and the cross-checking of planetary health knowledge.

This framework addresses the issue of the prevalent anthropocentric view that humans are the most significant beings on Earth. This is based on the notion that humans have always brought about significant changes to the world, such as the construction of landmarks and infrastructure. However, our planet was shaped by millions of functioning ecosystems that interacted with one another long before humans existed. All the resources we have exploited in the past and present are the result of these intricate yet delicate interactions. By clinging to the 'outdated' notion that humans are the sole agents of change on Earth, we adopt a naive and condescending posture, as we fail to recognise our dependence on these other biological systems. Conducting decision making at any level of government with a singular focus on human welfare is precisely what causes climate action efforts to be delayed and insufficient. Our sense of superiority over other sentient creatures leads to a lack of empathy and checks and balances in our approach to climate action. This relatively significant disconnection with the environment must and can be surmounted by implementing the governance framework for planetary health. The framework accentuates the need for us to expand and include other actors who play equally crucial roles in the surrounding ecosystems. To achieve this, we must first stop viewing human health as the only concern when it comes to environmental deterioration and begin contemplating the impacts on other forms of life (Ozdemir, 2019).

Winstead (2022) defines the Anthropocene as a perilous endeavour for humanity, as it threatens the delicate equilibrium between humans and animal life by invading the planetary boundaries of biodiversity. According to Winstead (2022) and Carrington (2017), the current rate of farming and urban planning has severe effects on migratory patterns, with knock-on effects on the animal food chain and human-dependent industries such as forestry and tourism. (Carrington, 2017) Changing migration patterns of disease-carrying organisms, such as malaria mosquitoes, has direct effects on public health hazards. The ongoing dispute between the United Kingdom, Iceland, and the Faroe Islands over mackerel allocation following the northern migration of the fish species exemplifies the centrality of this human–animal relationship in politics and international agreements (British Sea Fishing, 2012). We cannot afford to place the health of animals and other life forms second to our own (Ozdemir, 2019). Unhealthy ecosystems will ultimately have a negative impact on human health as well. Governance must therefore shape the public consensus on environmental issues to be more grounded in biodiversity and the sentience of other life forms on Earth. Recognising animal sentience will be a step in the correct direction for governance, as it will allow policymakers to gain a broader understanding of the interconnectedness of our ecosystems. Environmental policies will now abandon the anthropocentric perspective and recognise the interdependence of all ecosystems. This mental shift will go a long way towards supporting social change and attaining the objective of shifting from a public health perspective to a planetary health perspective.

In addition, the framework commits to deciphering the connection between politics and health. Planetary Health believes that there is a relationship between them and that we must be aware of these political determinants of health in governance. Despite appearing to be unrelated, health and power politics have an interactive relationship and, as highlighted in the preceding section, operate across all life forms (Ozdemir, 2019). This inseparability of knowledge and politics has inevitably led to bias in academic publications and influenced the implementation of policy. This inseparability must not, however, be a barrier to trust in governance; rather, it is an opportunity to include them in project planning. The importance of an interdisciplinary approach to environmental efforts is emphasised by planetary health (Ozdemir, 2019). The discipline of political science will play a crucial role in providing the necessary instruments and understanding of how social values and power struggles impact the decision-making process for climate action. This creates a more mature understanding of how systems function in this world, one that does not disregard human health. Now, medical specialists will collaborate with policy experts to propose environmental projects that include political risk assessments and decision-making process cross-checks. We cannot allow our historical ignorance of human and political influence in public health to prevent us from utilising this framework, which will ensure innovation is achieved bias-free.

Lastly, this governance framework also examines the potential political influences of addressing the proposed politics of planetary health. While attempting to resolve the relationship between science and politics, the question of how much we can trust the methodology used to study this relationship arises (Ozdemir, 2019). Can we trust the experts researching planetary health, and if not, how can we trust planetary health studies? These concerns must be posed to all decision-makers across all sectors and the scientific community, including planetary health researchers. Our previous discussions on reestablishing our relationship with the Earth's ecosystems surpassed the technical knowledge of planetary health and provided frameworks on how humanistic values influence health, encompassing knowledge of the social context. Now, the governance framework takes its third and final phase to emphasise knowledge-on-knowledge, posing epistemological questions like how do we know what we know (Ozdemir, 2019). This often-overlooked phase is crucial, as it relates to the veracity of prior environmental studies and ensures that biases do not exist in the very institutions battling them. As outlined in the preceding framework, cross-checks must be conducted even for planetary health regulators and expert committees, assessing their backgrounds and any potential sources of bias. Ozdemir proposes that planetary health be regarded as a knowledge ecosystem composed of protagonists (researchers working on technical knowledge) and narrators (research on research) in this framework. Such a viewpoint would be beneficial for those working on planetary health because it promotes the healthy practice of mutual cross-examination, thereby enhancing the credibility of academic publications. Educators of planetary health will now be more accountable and transparent in their work, fostering a positive academic atmosphere.

In conclusion, three essential areas of the governance framework for planetary health have been identified. We began with a discussion of the need and means to shift the perception of public health towards planetary health. In addition to highlighting the dangers of an anthropocentric view of planetary health, a proposal was made to recognise all life forms as equally essential and interdependent in one vast web of life. Then, we continued discussing the connection between science and politics. Both are not mutually exclusive and must be considered when making a decision. A multidisciplinary team would significantly benefit global health initiatives by assisting them in overcoming social barriers. The framework concludes with a reminder that biases can exist anywhere, including among the experts in planetary health who define the concept's course. To ensure a flourishing knowledge ecosystem, participants in planetary health are encouraged to perpetually assess and offer constructive criticism. It is anticipated that this framework will serve as a guide for improved governance and pave the way for the effective implementation of planetary health.

2.4 Challenges at the Global Level

Despite the evident advantages of adopting a planetary health approach as opposed to a traditional one, it still confronts potential threats that can be challenging to surmount. Climate change mitigation has never been simple, and this is especially true for the adoption of planetary health, which addresses the fundamental understanding of our relationship with Earth's ecosystems. Previous climate change initiatives focused on aspects of climate change mitigation and adaptation but struggled to garner support. Planetary health, on the other hand, addresses more crucial issues in environmental studies, such as the social influences of public health and the inherent biases in academic sources. Consequently, the welfare of the planet confronts a series of political issues.

Influencing political will to support the framework for planetary health will be a formidable obstacle among the problems it will confront. Initially, planetary health incorporates shifts in our past approaches to public health and the administration of a vast array of interconnected and complex ecosystems. The implementation of the various proposed frameworks will need to be discussed at the policymaking level, necessitating extensive research, lobbying, and other processes. Simply stated, the process requires significantly more energy and time than the alternative of using existing security systems. Furthermore, will planetary health still be valued when confronted with pressing economic and political issues? As proponents of planetary health confront a potential backlash from electors who doubt their posture, the problem of issue salience persists. This is particularly true for disadvantaged communities that are barely enduring their current economic and social difficulties. Man-made and natural disasters necessitate prompt action and difficult decisions from the government. Tragic events, such as the Russia-Ukraine War, resulted in widespread environmental devastation and population displacement. In light of geo-politics and survival, it may be difficult to locate a solid implementation platform for planetary health initiatives. In conclusion, effective implementation of planetary health requires a stable and politically willing government, which explains why green policies are prevalent in more developed nations. Considering the histori-cal context of environmental degradation and the economy over the past centuries, these more capable nations have an overarching obligation to lead planetary health initiatives and facilitate their incremental implementation for others.

In an attempt to create a more inclusive model, planetary health now confronts a problem of complexity that can potentially cause disorganisation in manage-ment. Among the defining characteristics of planetary health is its emphasis on cross-sector knowledge sharing, necessitating the formation of multidisciplinary teams. Their ability to collaborate on a common objective may be in question due to their diverse objectives and sectorial origins. Funding organisations for envi-ronmental initiatives may now be required to revise their policies, implementing planetary health significantly more complex than merely redefining public health. Disorganised planetary health management will only further risk it from being fa-voured in policymaking. Combined with the absence of unified global governance on planetary health, this impedes the implementation of the change and slows its progression. Drivers of environmental change will face a formidable challenge in achieving planetary health that is balanced between competing interests and pri-orities. Overall, the systems approach to planetary health results in new forms of challenges that public health may not have previously comprehensively consid-ered. Unquestionably, to form a framework that is more inclusive of multi-sector influences on health, the agents of this change must also be prepared to address the upcoming multi-sector challenges. Despite the inherent difficulty of these ob-stacles, they must not be a deterrent to the implementation of planetary health as better frameworks become readily available over time. Planetary health already recognises these potential dangers and provides adequate direction for overcoming them. Inter-disciplinary teams foster the knowledge-sharing necessary to confront these challenges head on. Consequently, new approaches to public health involve new challenges, but it is from these new challenges that new solutions emerge.

2.5 Conclusion

The concept of planetary health and its historical context have been emphasised throughout this paper. It was introduced to challenge the conventional approach to public health, which struggled to take adequate and punctual measures to combat environmental degradation. To date, climate action and health experts have neglected to address the primary upstream factors causing adverse health effects. We must recognise that previous research has been constrained by disciplinary boundaries and frequently ignored the influence of economic, political, and social forces on research outcomes and the subsequent implementation of policies. By believing that humans are the sole agents of change, we disregard that all biological systems are interconnected and ultimately affect human health. Planetary health believes that we must reconsider our place in the Earth's ecosystem and assume stewardship of its systems. Placing equal significance on all forms of existence will create a healthy environment for all individuals and beings. As it instils a sense of concern for our surrounding environment, addressing the effective aspects of education will be crucial to the success of planetary health education. Providing students with the historical and political context of the environment will produce a more knowledgeable and adaptable generation. Continuous cross-checking of proposed planetary health frameworks fosters a healthy knowledge ecosystem in the sciences that aspires for gradual development.

Planetary health encounters several obstacles that may impede its implementation on a global scale. At its foundation, planetary health confronts these obstacles because it necessitates profound shifts in human behaviour and outlook. To garner political support from policymakers, it would be necessary to develop robust and organised frameworks for planetary health that address the issues of complexity and salience. Environmental education will require revisions, and educators must support efforts to inculcate in people a larger sense of long-term value. In the same way that the challenges of planetary health are multifaceted, their solutions are of a similar character and require knowledge and experience in a variety of fields. Despite these ostensibly formidable obstacles, embracing planetary health cannot be considered unimportant, as it is essential to our long-term survival. Ignoring it will only result in a continued misunderstanding of our planet's ecosystems and, consequently, ineffective climate action. As evidenced throughout this text, proponents of planetary health have already begun proposing frameworks and presenting the public with their potential benefits. These efforts must be shared with the general public to garner additional support for their eventual intragovernmental and international implementation. It is anticipated that users of planetary health will incorporate these modifications into their decision-making and uphold them at all levels of decision-making. The positive knowledge ecosystem of planetary health encourages solutions to be continually evaluated and reevaluated over time, leaving future generations better prepared for environmental survival.

References

British Sea Fishing. (2012, July 19). *Mackerel War | British Sea Fishing*. British Sea Fishing. https://britishseafishing.co.uk/the-mackerel-wars/

Bromley-Trujillo, R., & Poe, J. (2018). The importance of salience: Public opinion and state policy action on climate change. *Journal of Public Policy*, *40*(2), 280–304. Cambridge Core. https://doi.org/10.1017/s0143814x18000375

Carrington, D. (2017, March 30). Climate change: Global reshuffle of wildlife will have huge impacts on humanity. *The Guardian*. https://www.theguardian.com/environment/2017/mar/30/climate-change-global-reshuffle-of-wildlife-will-have-huge-impacts-on-humanity#:~:text=The%20most%20direct%20impact%20on

Crawley, S., Coffé, H., & Chapman, R. (2019). Public opinion on climate change: Belief and concern, issue salience and support for government action. *The British Journal of Politics and International Relations*, *22*(1), 102–121. https://doi.org/10.1177/1369148119888827

Crawley, S., Coffé, H., & Chapman, R. (2021). Climate belief and issue salience: Comparing two dimensions of public opinion on climate change in the EU. *Social Indicators Research*, *162*, 307–325. https://doi.org/10.1007/s11205-021-02842-0

Dabla-Norris, E., Helbling, T., Khalid, S., Khan, H., Magistretti, G., Sollaci, A., & Srinivasan, K. (2023). *Public perceptions of climate mitigation policies*. International Monetary Fund.

Gabrys, J. (2020). Planetary health in practice: Sensing air pollution and transforming urban environments. *Humanities and Social Sciences Communications*, *7*(1), 1–10. https://doi.org/10.1057/s41599-020-00534-7

Guzmán, C. A. F., Aguirre, A. A., Astle, B., Barros, E., Bayles, B., Chimbari, M., El-Abbadi, N., Evert, J., Hackett, F., Howard, C., Jennings, J., Krzyzek, A., LeClair, J., Maric, F., Martin, O., Osano, O., Patz, J., Potter, T., Redvers, N., & Trienekens, N. (2021). A framework to guide planetary health education. *The Lancet Planetary Health*, *5*(5), e253–e255. https://doi.org/10.1016/s2542-5196(21)00110-8

Heilmayr, R., Echeverría, C., & Lambin, E. F. (2020). Impacts of Chilean forest subsidies on forest cover, carbon and biodiversity. *Nature Sustainability*, *3*(9), 701–709. Springer Nature. https://doi.org/10.1038/s41893-020-0547-0

Horton, R., Beaglehole, R., Bonita, R., Raeburn, J., McKee, M., & Wall, S. (2014). From public to planetary health: A manifesto. *The Lancet Planetary Health*, *383*, 847.

Horton, R., & Lo, S. (2015). Planetary health: A new science for exceptional action. *The Lancet*, *386*, 1921–1922.

Khan, A., Mojumder, S. K., Kovats, S., & Vineis, P. (2008). Saline contamination of drinking water in Bangladesh. *The Lancet*, *371*(9610), 385. https://doi.org/10.1016/s0140-6736(08)60197-x

Myers, S. S. (2017). Planetary health: Protecting human health on a rapidly changing planet. *The Lancet*, *390*, 2860–2868.

Özdemir, V. (2019). Innovating governance for planetary health with three critically informed frames. *OMICS: A Journal of Integrative Biology*, *23*(12), 623–630. https://doi.org/10.1089/omi.2019.0175

Planetary Health Alliance. (2023). *Planetary health*. Retrieved September 15, 2023, from https://www.planetaryhealthalliance.org/planetary-health

Planetary Health Alliance. (2015). *About PHA - Planetary health alliance*. https://www.planetaryhealthalliance.org/about-pha

Pongsiri, M. J., Gatzweiler, F. W., Bassi, A. M., Haines, A., & Demassieux, F. (2017). The need for a systems approach to planetary health. *The Lancet Planetary Health*, *1*(7), e257–e259. https://doi.org/10.1016/s2542-5196(17)30116-x

Saier, A. (2022, October 24). *Climate plans remain insufficient: More ambitious action needed now*. United Nations Climate Change. https://unfccc.int/news/climate-plans-remain-insufficient-more-ambitious-action-needed-now#:~:text=We%20are%20still%20nowhere%20near

Spisak, B. R., State, B., van de Leemput, I., Scheffer, M., & Liu, Y. (2022). Large-scale decrease in the social salience of climate change during the COVID-19 pandemic. *PLoS One*, *17*(1), 1–6. https://doi.org/10.1371/journal.pone.0256082

Stantcheva, S. (2024, January 19). *How communication helps translate climate policies into action*. World Economic Forum. https://www.weforum.org/stories/2024/01/people-are-worried-about-climate-change-but-still-don-t-take-action-recent-research-explains-why/

Thompson, A. (2021, June 30). *Revealed: ExxonMobil's lobbying war on climate change legislation*. Channel 4 News. https://www.channel4.com/news/revealed-exxonmobils-lobbying-war-on-climate-change-legislation#:~:text=In%20the%20excerpts%20from%20the

Tranter, B., Lester, L., Foxwell-Norton, K., & Palmer, M. A. (2023). In science we trust? Public trust in intergovernmental panel on climate change projections and accepting anthropogenic climate change. *Public Understanding of Science*, *32*(6), 096366252311654. https://doi.org/10.1177/09636625231165405

US EPA. (2014, April 17). *Economics of biofuels*. https://www.epa.gov/environmental-economics/economics-biofuels#:~:text=Regarding%20non%2DGHG%20environmental%20impacts

Winstead, A. (2022, April 20). *Humans and animal migration: A complex and interwoven issue*. Unsustainable Magazine. https://www.unsustainablemagazine.com/humans-and-animal-migration/

3

WESTERN COMMITMENT
TO PLANETARY HEALTH

John Harrison and Immanuel Azaad Moonesar

3.1 Introduction

Human health is generally better today than it has ever been. In 1950–1955, life expectancy was 47 years; in 2005–2010, it was 69 years. As a result of ignoring the long-term effects of human activity on the natural processes on our planet, our ability to offer health care to those in need has been severely disrupted. A global pandemic of the unique SARSCOV-2 virus, which had been projected for some time due to shifting land-use patterns, growing urbanization, natural evolution, climate change, and human intrusion into formerly pristine areas, has claimed the lives of more than five million people (Dong et al., 2020; Iyer et al., 2021).

"Our planet, our health" was the topic of 2024. World Health Day, which fell on April 7. The health of the Earth and the health of its inhabitants are interdependent. Increased use and reliance on fossil fuels are responsible for an estimated 13 million fatalities each year, with the number predicted to climb if current habits are not changed. World Health Day served as a timely and vital warning that global crises are intertwined with climate change and that we must not lose sight of the existential threat that ecological degradation offers to planetary and human health (The Lancet Public Health, 2022).

Planetary Health is referred to as the *"field of study that aims to produce knowledge regarding relationships between human activities, their impacts on environment and downstream consequences to health of humans, other living organisms, and natural systems"* (Myers & Frumkin, 2020).

3.1.1 Formulation of Planetary Health

When applied to natural systems, this formulation presents a conceptual framework for appreciating the linkages between human health and natural systems at

DOI: 10.4324/9781003569084-4

the systems level. The concept of planetary health is similar to eco-social theories of causation in that it integrates human health into a system that explicitly accounts for biological, social, and environmental factors, similar to the Social-Ecological Systems theory. Interrelationships between human health, environmental health, and underlying socioeconomic situations are all investigated by researchers, and each has an impact on the others. Furthermore, planetary health researches how human actions affect the health of natural systems and vice versa in order to prevent global warming. From both a human and a natural systems perspective, it becomes clear that human health is dependent on the health of natural systems that provide the basic ecosystem services that enable food production, clean water and air, and recreational space, among other things.

After the Rockefeller–Lancet Commission Report was published in 2015, it inspired the creation of a new academic field called planetary health as a reaction to the world's ongoing environmental problems and crises (Whitmee et al., 2015). Medical ecologists established this field decades ago, and Indigenous societies have long held the belief that human health and the natural environment are interwoven, as do medical ecologists. The growth of planetary health as an academic effort, as a result, acts as an umbrella to bring scientists and politicians together around a common issue and influence research agendas advocated by varied alliances. As a result of this deliberate effort to include opinions from a diverse range of scientific domains, experts from various disciplines can lend their support to the project. It is a top goal for practitioners to understand how social systems influence the planet's health, and social scientists are invited to contribute to this understanding (Iyer et al., 2021). To ensure global well-being, it is necessary to do in-depth research into the relationship between human economic activity and the evolution of Earth's systems. It is feasible to find solutions to problems that appear intractable from a single scientific area perspective. When evidence from a range of disciplines is used to support a policy, the case for the policy becomes more powerful.

3.1.1.1 *Trends and Drivers in Global Environmental Change*

The SARS-COV-2 pandemic (Covid-19), which was a rare but devastating external shock, highlighted the vulnerability of our highly controlled economic and health systems by the severity of the human and socioeconomic effects. At the same time, climate change, freshwater resources, ocean acidification, changes in land use and soil erosion, nitrogen and phosphorus pollution, toxic chemical pollution and exposure, biodiversity loss, and other trends in global environmental change are all being addressed, not to mention the factors and drivers of environmental change such as population growth, consumption, and technological advancement (Whitmee et al., 2015).

A deterioration in the quality of ecosystem services (which refers to the advantages to humans provided by healthy ecosystems) has been recorded worldwide, according to the planetary health community. Environmental scientists, physicians, and public health practitioners have all reported this decline (Myers & Frumkin, 2020). According to the "Great Acceleration" theory proposed by Steffen and colleagues, human populations and economic activities are changing at the same rate as the planet's systems are changing. As a result of mounting evidence that human activities are deteriorating the Earth's systems, the Planetary Boundaries concept was established to establish environmental degradation thresholds for use in future research and development. According to the Planetary Boundaries theory, exceeding certain environmental degradation thresholds would have catastrophic consequences for both human health and the health of natural systems on the planet (Iyer et al., 2021). Earlier this year, the Intergovernmental Science-Policy Platform on Biodiversity and Ecosystem Services (IPBES) reported that ecosystem declines have been accelerating in recent decades, with 47% declines in ecosystem extent and condition, 82% declines in biomass and species abundance, and 25% of species threatened with extinction (Diaz et al., 2019). The deforestation and desertification of the world's forests and deserts (as well as the loss of wetlands and biodiversity) are examples of human-induced strain on natural systems that cannot be sustained. Other examples are the depletion of freshwater resources and urbanization.

Environmental and planetary health professionals used public health and epidemiology research to assess the long-term threats to humans posed by the degradation of natural systems and to identify strategies for reducing poor health outcomes (Myers & Frumkin, 2020). The health of humans is affected both directly and indirectly by changes in natural systems at the macro scale. Higher floods, more severe heat waves, and pollution exposure are all direct health concerns, but livelihoods are threatened, and people are forced to flee their homes, which constitutes indirect health risks (Whitmee et al., 2015).

According to planetary health studies, the acts of humans may have long-term consequences for human well-being. Although some of these changes to natural systems, such as land use and urbanization, are associated with significant risks to the environment, they have historically been justified to enhance human health in the short term through economic development (Iyer et al., 2021). As part of our efforts to achieve global development goals, such as the Sustainable Development Goals 2030, which call for increased economic growth to promote health and social well-being, we may need to change our energy and nutritional habits (United Nations, 2015). During this section, you will learn about a systems-oriented approach that was established by Planetary Health to link human progress with environmental deterioration and human health.

3.1.2   Policies in Public Health

Policies in public health that have a positive impact on both human health and the environment are referred to as "win-win" policies.

3.1.2.1 Emissions of Greenhouse Gases on the Rise

When actions taken to reduce greenhouse gas emissions in the housing, transportation, food and agriculture, and electricity generation sectors result in health benefits, this is referred to as co-benefits. These advantages are frequently significant in nature. It is paramount to note that one of the mechanisms is the reduction of fine-particle air pollution, which is an important mechanism. In each year, between 28,000 and 36,000 people die as a result of ambient air pollution from fine particulates, depending on where the pollution comes from. Carbon dioxide emissions from the combustion of fossil fuels, particularly coal and diesel fuel, are responsible for the vast majority of these deaths (Lim et al., 2012). The World Health Organization estimates that 37 million people will die in 2012, which is an increase from the previous year's estimates (WHO, 2014). Reducing fine-particulate air pollution as a result of reduced fossil fuel combustion has been extensively researched, and the evidence has been compiled by the Intergovernmental Panel on Climate Change and the Lancet Commission on Climate Change, among others (IPCC, 2014; Whitmee et al., 2015). It is not necessary to discuss these advantages in detail in this report because they have already been summarized elsewhere.

3.1.2.2 Pollutants with a Short Half-Life in the Environment

It is estimated that some measures to reduce black carbon exposure could prevent an estimated 24.4 million premature deaths per year around the world as a result of the reduction of short-lived climate pollutants. As a result, some efforts to reduce short-lived climate pollutants also result in reductions in carbon dioxide emissions, which increases the overall effectiveness of climate-change initiatives (Shindell et al., 2012). The use of clean energy by households has the potential to reduce their exposure to air pollution, the risk of fire, and the emissions of black carbon and a variety of other polluting pollutants, among other things (Afrane et al., 2022). In the case of solar lamps, for example, they can assist in reducing black carbon emissions, burns, and the reliance on expensive kerosene by as much as 50%.

The reduction of ground-level ozone, which results from chemical reactions between nitrogen oxides, methane, and volatile organic compounds, can have co-benefits in addition to their primary purpose of reducing air pollution. Reduced ground-level ozone can be beneficial in a variety of ways. Besides having a negative impact on human health, ozone air pollution also has a detrimental effect on crop productivity, forest growth, and the ability of vegetation to absorb carbon dioxide from the atmosphere (Abduljabbar et al., 2021). Decreased crop productivity, as a result of lower tropospheric ozone levels, has been shown to be associated with improved human health and increased agricultural productivity as a result of policies to reduce methane emissions.

3.1.2.3 Increased Physical Activity

Walking and cycling more frequently in cities can help to reduce greenhouse gas and fine particulate emissions while also combating physical inactivity, which is responsible for more than 3 million deaths per year (Lim et al., 2012) and is a risk factor for major noncommunicable diseases such as ischaemic heart disease, stroke, diabetes, colon and breast cancer, Alzheimer's disease, and other mental illnesses. It is generally agreed that the health benefits outweigh the increased risk of road injuries in most cases. Although they may reduce hazardous pollutants emitted from tailpipes, new technologies such as electric vehicles will not address other public health issues such as physical inactivity or road accidents, according to the World Health Organization. Further research has found that obesity is associated with increased physical activity related to transportation and changes in dietary habits (Tilman & Clark, 2014). Obesity could potentially be addressed by strategies that reduce the use of private automobiles in metropolitan areas, such as improving public transportation and encouraging active travel, by improving public transportation and encouraging active travel.

References

Abduljabbar, R. L., Liyanage, S., & Dia, H. (2021). The role of micro-mobility in shaping sustainable cities: A systematic literature review. *Transportation Research Part D: Transport and Environment, 92,* 102734.

Afrane, S., Ampah, J. D., & Mensah, E. A. (2022). Visualization and analysis of mapping knowledge domains for the global transition towards clean cooking: A bibliometric review of research output from 1990 to 2020. *Environmental Science and Pollution Research, 29*(16), 23041–23068.

Diaz, S., Settele, E., Brondizio, E., Nguo, H., Gueze, M., Agard, J., Arneth, A., Balvanera, P., Brauman, K. A., Butchart, S. H. M., Chan, K. M. A., Garibaldi, L. A., Liu, K. I. J., Subramanian, S. M., Midgley, G. F., Miloslavich, P., Molnár, Z., Obura, D., Pfaff, A., … Zayas, C. N. (2019). *Summary for policymakers of the global assessment report on biodiversity and ecosystem services of the intergovernmental science-policy* (Version 1). IPBES. https://doi.org/10.5281/zenodo.3553458

Dong, E., Du, H., & Gardner, L. (2020). An interactive web-based dashboard to track COVID-19 in real-time. *The Lancet Infectious Diseases, Elsevier, 20*(5), 533–534.

IPCC. (2014). Climate change 2014: Impacts, adaptation, and vulnerability – IPCC WGII AR5 summary for policymakers. In C. B. Field, V. R. Barros, D. J. Dokken, K. J. Mach, M. D. Mastrandrea, T. E. Bilir, M. Chatterjee, K. L. Ebi, Y. O. Estrada, R. C. Genova, B. Girma, E. S. Kissel, A. N. Levy, S. MacCracken, P. R. Mastrandrea, & L. L. White (Eds.), *Climate change 2014: Impacts, adaptation, and vulnerability. Part A: Global and sectoral aspects. Contribution of working group II to the fifth assessment report of the intergovernmental panel on climate change* (pp. 1–32). Cambridge University Press.

Iyer, H. S., DeVille, N. V., Stoddard, O., Cole, J., Myers, S. S., Li, H., Elliott, E. G., Jimenez, M., James, P., & Golden, P. (2021). Sustaining planetary health through systems thinking: Public health's critical role. *SSM-Population Health, 15,* 100844.

Lim, S. S., Vos, T., Flaxman, A. D., Danaei, G., Shibuya, K., Adair-Rohani, H., AlMazroa, M. A., Amann, M., Ross Anderson, H., Andrews, K. G., Aryee, M., Atkinson, C., Bacchus, L. J., Bahalim, A. N., Balakrishnan, K., Balmes, J., Barker-Collo, S., Baxter, A., Bell, M. L., … Ezzati, M. (2012). A comparative risk assessment of burden of disease and injury attributable to 67 risk factors and risk factor clusters in 21 regions, 1990–2010: A systematic analysis for the Global Burden of Disease Study 2010. *The Lancet, 380*, 2224–2260.

Myers, S., & Frumkin, H. (2020). *Planetary health: Protecting nature to protect ourselves.* Island Press.

Shindell, D., Kuylenstierna, J. C., Vignati, E., van Dingenen, R., Amann, M., Klimont, Z., Anenberg, S. C., Muller, N., Janssens-Maenhout, G., Raes, F., Schwartz, J., Faluvegi, G., Pozzoli, L., Kupiainen, K., Höglund-Isaksson, L., Emberson, L., Streets, D., Ramanathan, V., Hicks, K., … Fowler, D. (2012). Simultaneously mitigating near-term climate change and improving human health and food security. *Science, 335*, 183–189.

The Lancet Public Health. (2022). No public health without planetary health. *The Lancet Public Health, 7*(4), e291. https://doi.org/10.1016/S2468-2667(22)00068-8

Tilman, D., & Clark, M. (2014). Global diets link environmental sustainability and human health. *Nature, 515*, 518–522.

United Nations. (2015). Transforming our world: The 2030 Agenda for sustainable development, No. A/RES/70/1. United Nations, New York, available at https://www.un.org/ga/search/view_doc.asp?symbol=A/RES/70/1&Lang=E

Whitmee, S., Haines, A., Beyrer, C., Boltz, F., Capon, A. G., de Souza Dias, B. F., Ezeh, A., Frumkin, H., Gong, P., Head, P., Horton, R., Mace, G. M., Marten, R., Myers, S. S., Nishtar, S., Osofsky, S. A., Pattanayak, S. K., Pongsiri, M. J., Romanelli, C., … Yach, D. (2015). Safeguarding human health in the Anthropocene epoch: Report of the Rockefeller foundation–lancet commission on planetary health. *The Lancet, 386*(10007), 1973–2028.

WHO. (2014). *7 million premature deaths annually linked to air pollution.* World Health Organization.

4

COVID-19 IN THE HIMALAYAN REGION

State Capacity and Non-Traditional Security Challenges

Joshua Snider[1]

4.1 Introduction

The COVID-19 pandemic is without question the most significant and most severe global public health crisis in the past century. The depth and severity of the crisis can be understood at the inter-state and intra-state levels. At the inter-state level, pandemic-driven border closures disrupted tourism travel trade, which had knock-on effects at the sub-state level in terms of food, energy, and societal security. At the intra-state level, the pandemic's toll can be measured by the loss of life, the impact on public health systems, and disruptions to education and the economy. The pandemic was a perfect storm for lower- and middle-income states generally. In the Indo-Pacific region, dynamics such as low state capacity, weak and under-funded public health systems, limited social welfare programs, ethno-religious populism, and low trust in governments, combined with demographic factors such as high-density living, multi-generational families, and transient and mobile populations all conspired to create an uncontrollable situation in respect to states' governance of the COVID-19 pandemic.

Amidst the pandemic's catastrophic impact on large states in the Indo-Pacific, there has been comparatively little focus on the pandemic's impact on smaller states and sub-regions. Moreover, the economic precarity of large peasant populations reliant on subsistence wages meant that states did not have the option to enact long-term lockdowns, nor did they have the resources to keep large and vulnerable populations out of poverty. Indeed, pandemic-driven precarity will be a structural challenge for lower- and middle-income states across the Indo-Pacific for decades to come.

Within an Indo-Pacific regional context, there has been comparatively little scholarly or media attention to the impact of, and response to, the pandemic in

DOI: 10.4324/9781003569084-5

the core Himalayan region.[2] This region is ethnically, culturally, and religiously diverse and stands at the geographic border between South and East Asia. The region is home to a variety of geopolitical entities and, for our purposes includes sovereign states, such as Bhutan, Nepal, and Indian union territories (Ladakh and Sikkim), and China (Tibet). It hosts bisecting nodes of geostrategic competition between multiple regional powers, primarily between China and India and between India and Pakistan (Aroor, 2021; Bhonsale, 2020). The geopolitical contestation plays out simultaneously at both inter- and intra-state levels and impacts trajectories of local politics.

The dynamics associated with the COVID-19 pandemic in this region exposed the capacity issues faced by low-income states in dealing with public health crises and the broader geostrategic challenge faced by states steering a middle path between regional power rivals. Regarding the pandemic itself, dynamics within the region presented similarities and differences. States within the region faced similar challenges in that all are mountainous with remote and isolated communities with limited and/or non-existent quarantine facilities. All have limited ICU facilities and a severe shortage of medical equipment needed to treat critically ill COVID-19 patients, notably ventilators. All states in the region also face doctor shortages, with Bhutan having the lowest per capita doctor-to-patient rates globally (Drexler, 2021a). However, beyond these structural similarities, the impact of, and response to, the pandemic played out differently within the region. On the one hand, Bhutan's response has been lauded as an example of efficiency and effective governance, especially given its very low capacity. Conversely, Nepal's response has been less effective and negatively impacted by numerous factors, ranging from planning to the under-funded public health system to dynamics associated with its geography.

For practitioners and scholars interested in the governance of non-traditional security (NTS) issues, the pandemic in the Himalayas presents a critical case. The scale and impact of the pandemic supports claim long made by NTS analysts and scholars that security studies has undergone a conceptual expansion to include non-military threats and challenges. Rather than being understood in narrowly statist terms (i.e., where security is achieved if states can repel external invasion or internal political challenge), security studies have grown to include various "referent objects," notably individuals and communities (Anthony et al., 2017). Thus, while states remain security managers, they deliver security outcomes to various constituencies, including the provision of societal goods in NTS sectors, including health, education, energy, the economy, and the environment. While states in the Global South generally struggle with capacity issues that impact outcomes in all NTS sectors, the COVID-19 pandemic has made providing outcomes in NTS sectors even more challenging.

While there has been considerable discussion about the pandemic and its impact on various parts of South and East Asia, the pandemic, and the response of states in the Himalayan region have been under-served by media and scholarly discourses alike. This chapter addresses this gap by examining the responses of three states in the core Himalayan region (Nepal, Bhutan, and Indian union territory of Ladakh) to the COVID-19 pandemic. The first section examines the initial outbreak and its impact on the three territories and analyses the scale of the outbreak in these states. The second section analyses response and containment measures undertaken by states, examining both direct public health responses and ancillary measures such as lockdowns and movement restrictions. The third section examines vaccination strategies, specifically how states secured doses and then rolled out vaccination programs. The final section examines the impact of the pandemic on NTS sectors beyond the public health crisis in areas related to economic security, social cohesion, and food security. All of this is offered to demonstrate that the pandemic's trajectory in the Himalayan region challenges assumptions about the capacity of small, low-capacity states to respond to a once-in-a-century public health crisis and "siloed approaches" to the governance of NTS. In this case, it is evident that a catastrophic deterioration in one NTS sector (health) significantly impacts others. This chapter evaluates the trajectory of the COVID-19 pandemic and state responses therein between January of 2020 and December of 2021, but it does not address the impact of the emerging Omicron variant.

4.2   Part 1: Outbreak and Infection

At a global level, the initial spread of COVID-19 reflected a mix of dynamics. Initially, the most significant issue was travel from the initial epicentre of the outbreak (Wuhan province) to the rest of the world. In its first wave, the spread of the virus was driven by travel. It occurred via the comingling of Chinese and North American tourists in southern Europe, which resulted in pandemics in North America and Europe. Consequently, the first wave of the pandemic more severely impacted southern Europe and North America. For example, the unwillingness of the Trump administration to shut US borders early and set up an effective testing regime exacerbated the rate of infection, which led to wide-scale community spread. Moreover, in Canada, the first wave of cases was driven by travel to Europe combined with winter travel to the southern United States. Transmission from the epicentres in China and Europe to Asia was facilitated by several factors, including the return of migrant labour from Arabian Gulf states to South Asia, returning South Asian students, and, to a lesser degree, tourism. In the initial phase of the pandemic, a widely circulated thesis argued that the COVID-19 pandemic would be a pandemic of the wealthy and old and thus would have a much bigger impact on Global North and or highly globalized societies and or old/aging societies like those in southern Europe. According to this argument, despite the limited public health capacity, the pandemic would be less severe in the Global South (Mukherjee, 2021). As we now know, while this argument was true to some extent in the first wave, it proved less accurate as the pandemic shifted from one driven by international travel to one driven by wide-scale community transmission. Moreover, while older people are more likely to experience more severe forms of the disease, younger people get infected at similar rates and are more likely to be asymptomatic. Of the four main variants, three have originated in Asia and Africa, including the most recent Omicron variant.

At the Himalayan regional level, overall trajectory of the pandemic in its initial phase was driven by a confluence of the region's under-development and limited public health capacity on the one hand and its proximity to China on the other (Channel News Asia, 2021). On a practical level, various arguments were offered to explain how the outbreak might unfold. For example, some argued that the initial phase might be catastrophic due to the region's proximity to the initial epicentre of the pandemic, China. Others argued that high elevation would provide a natural level of protection against the virus (Indian Express, 2020). Both of these arguments proved to be partially true. While it is true that the Himalayan region saw large-scale infections, high death rates and wide disruption to social and economic life, neither the proximity to China nor the high altitude fully explained transmission and or infection or death rates (ICIMOD, 2020). The analysis in the remainder of this section will assess the scale of the COVID-19 outbreak in Nepal, Bhutan, and Ladakh. least.

4.2.1 Nepal

Given that Nepal is the largest of the Himalayan states (with a population of 29 million), and it is the most globalized in terms both of tourism and outbound travel amongst Nepalese, it stands to reason that the pandemic has been more acute than in neighbouring Bhutan or India's Himalayan territories. According to Nepal's Ministry of Health and Population (MoHP) and the World Health Organization (WHO), as of 2 January 2022, the country had confirmed 827,972 cases, 798,916 recoveries, and 11,590 deaths ("Nepal: WHO Coronavirus Disease (COVID-19) Dashboard With Vaccination Data", 2022). The most significant spike in cases occurred between April and September of 2021, when cases averaged between 8000 and 9000 per day, coinciding with the worst Delta wave in India. In May of 2021, Nepal had the highest average infection rate in the world (Callamard, 2021). During this wave the dynamics in Nepal were, by most accounts, very similar to India's in terms of the lack of capacity in the public health system to cope with hospitalizations and lack of personal protective equipment (PPE) and oxygen tanks. Between 2020 to 2021 public health authorities performed 4,530,686 polymerase chain reaction (PCR) tests and set up a testing regime that included 40 dedicated laboratories (Government of Nepal, 2021).

Nepal's first case (also the first in South Asia) was detected on 23 January 2020, following the return of a 31-year-old man who had been studying in Wuhan (Chalise, 2020). Thereafter, Nepal's first incident of local transmission occurred on 4 April and its first fatality occurred on 14 May (Chalise, 2020). Since then, the virus has been detected in all country regions, with heavily populated Bagmati and Kathmandu provinces and districts being the most heavily impacted. Unlike other

Himalayan states, Nepal exports many labourers to Southeast Asia and the Arabian Gulf regions (Neuman, 2021). While the rate of infection amongst repatriated Nepalese nationals has been not disaggregated from the overall numbers, repatriated nationals likely contributed to the initial trajectory of spread. Amidst economic disruption in the ASEAN and Gulf regions in the first wave of the pandemic, many Nepalese were repatriated. It is unclear how many of the repatriated Nepalese workers came back ill or contracted the virus in transit and thus contributed to the pandemic's outcome at a local level once home. According to the Non-Resident Nepali Association, as of 26 July 2020, there were a total of 12,667 confirmed cases, 16,190 recoveries, and 161 deaths across 35 countries (Neuman, 2021).

4.2.2 Bhutan

The Kingdom of Bhutan is an isolated, semi-sovereign state with a population of 770,000. Unlike Nepal, it has comparatively low outward migration rates amongst its local population and a burgeoning but small tourism industry. According to the WHO, as of 2 January 2022, the country had had 2660 COVID-19 cases and three deaths (Reuters, 2021). The most significant spike in cases occurred between March and July of 2021, when cases averaged between 100 and 200 per day, coinciding with the worst Delta wave in India (Reuters). Also, Bhutan's reported case fatality rate of 0.05% compares very favourably to the WHO's reported global fatality rates, which stand at 4.34% (Bhaduri, 2021).

There has been no community transmission of COVID-19 in Bhutan, with all cases originating from overseas travel. The country's first confirmed cases occurred on 6 March 2020, when two elderly American tourists from India tested positive. Between March and June of 2020, there was limited community spread, and the trajectory of infection was confined to the return of small numbers of expatriate Bhutanese (Tamang & Dorji, 2021). While Bhutan does not have a large expatriate migrant workforce by South Asian standards, a vast majority of the infection was transmitted by Bhutanese travellers originating from the Arabian Gulf region, and to a lesser degree returning Bhutanese students who were studying in the US and UK (Tamang & Dorji, 2021). Given the small numbers and limited entry points to the country, the state was able to quarantine inbound passengers.

4.2.3 Ladakh

The Indian union territory of Ladakh (UT) has a population of 247,000 and has undergone significant changes over the past two years (2021–2022). Between 1947 and 2019, it was part of Jammu and Kashmir's Muslim majority union territory. In 2019, the Territory of Jammu and Kashmir was partitioned into two union territories, Jammu and Kashmir, and Ladakh (Aroor, 2021). The former has a majority Muslim population, whereas the latter has a majority Buddhist population. By most accounts, the partition was popular, and there is a high level of satisfaction and trust amongst Ladakhis with the Indian state. According to the WHO, as of 29 December 2021, the territory had had 22,140 COVID-19 cases, 21,707 recoveries, and 219 deaths (Rehman et al., 2020). A vast majority of the cases were in the UT's two main population centres, Leh and Kargil. Like the other states in the region, the most significant spike in cases occurred between March and July of 2021, coinciding with the worst Delta wave in India (Rehman et al., 2020). Given Ladakh's integration into India, there is little disaggregated data on the extent of the pandemic as data is often combined with West Bengal (Aroor, 2021). As such, there is no data on the relative infection or death rate in Ladakh.

Ladakh's first case was reported on 7 March 2020, when two Ladakhi pilgrims returned from Iran with COVID-19 symptoms. On 17 March, another case was detected from a known associate of one of the pilgrims. It seems that through aggressive lockdowns and contact tracing, the UT government was able to prevent large-scale community transmission of the virus. That said, at the height of the Delta wave, which had a disproportionate effect on India, it became more difficult for the UT government to prevent community transmissions. Consequently, for six months (starting in March of 2021), Ladakh's daily case rates went from 0 to 50–70 per day (Rehman et al., 2020). At the end of 2021, there was another spike from 35 cases in the week ending 27 October 2021 to 157 cases in the week ending 17 November 2021 (Rehman et al., 2020).

While population density in Nepal, Bhutan, and Ladakh are low by South Asian standards, a major possibly complicating factor that could have impacted the infection trajectory was many Buddhist monasteries in the region. This fact posed its challenges in a) moderating communal religious activities and b) the general communal living conditions within the monastic communities. Despite initial concerns that monasteries could be "super spreader" environments, the data suggests this was not the case. No studies have been undertaken to examine how monastic communities in either territory reacted to the pandemic. However, anecdotally it seems that monastic leadership worked efficiently with governments and put in place measures to ensure that monasteries did not become sites of significant transmission.

The analysis in this section has discussed the initial spread of the COVID-19 virus in the Himalayan region. To this end, we see that states in the region present divergent internal dynamics regarding the spread of the virus. Like elsewhere, the initial arrival of the virus was due to travel – from China (in the case of Nepal), from India (in the case of Bhutan), and Iran (in the case of Ladakh). As previously noted, the spread of the virus varied greatly between states in the region. Nepal had to reintegrate many returning expatriate workers, while Ladakh and Bhutan host large monastic communities. Nepal is the largest state in the region and had the highest rates of community spread and a high death rate. Equating the trajectories of transmission with levels of development is problematic. While Nepal is objectively "more developed" than Bhutan, the former has suffered much worse outcomes. In contrast, Bhutan has an objectively less developed public health system than Nepal but has suffered less severe consequences in terms of overall infection and death rates. Thus, smaller and more isolated states (Bhutan and Ladakh) have had comparatively low death rates and limited community spread.

4.3 Part 2: Response and Containment Measures

In the context of a global pandemic, containment measures address two different but inter-related problems: preventing community spread while preventing new cases entering from overseas. While states were unable to stop the initial spread of the COVID-19 virus, the question quickly turned to containment (i.e., how best to mitigate the worst possible scenarios). Unlike the 2003 SARS virus, which had a high death rate but was not particularly infectious, the Sars-COV-2 variant has a very high transmissibility rate, which stymied efforts to contain the virus and prevent large-scale community transmission (CDC, 2022). Thus, the COVID-19 pandemic quickly became a "transnational" public health crisis to the extent that it spread within and between countries. Containment responses to the pandemic included public health measures such as mask mandates, testing, contact tracing, and quarantines and public order measures such as police-enforced lockdowns, curfews, internal mobility restriction, and international border closures. These measures set off intense debates within many states on the state's right to limit movement in the name of public health, the impact of economic disruption born from lockdowns, and the extent to which the proverbial cure (i.e., containment measures) might be worse than the disease ("COVID-19 LSE Research", 2022). In the first instance, questions were raised regarding the overall aim of the containment measure, i.e., to completely obliterate the virus or to manage its spread to a reasonable degree? States such as China, Australia, New Zealand, and parts of Asia maintained versions of "zero COVID-19 strategies" to completely eradicate the virus (Syailendrawati et al., 2022). This strategy entailed aggressive lockdowns and border closures. Other states, particularly those in the Middle East, Western Europe, and the US, saw this as impractical and instead tried to contain the spread of the virus while achieving a level of normalcy (Syailendrawati et al., 2022). In addition, questions were raised about the efficacy of various public health approaches in mask mandates and venue closures.

Given the long duration of the COVID-19 pandemic, containment measures have evolved significantly in most states. In the first pandemic wave when there were no treatments or viable vaccines, the only responses were mitigation measures to "circuit break" cycles of community transmission through movement limitations and quarantine. As the pandemic went on, most states moved away from zero COVID-19 strategies and used various means to control infection rates when numbers hit certain levels, thus applying restrictions selectively as infections rates rise and fall. Moreover, from late 2020 until the onset of the Omicron variant in late 2021, many states moved away from aggressive containment strategies (in the form of lockdowns and movement restrictions) towards more flexible measures.

Thus, there was broad agreement that eradication was not a practical goal. Therefore, accepting a certain level of COVID-19 in communities was the price to be paid for opening economies and borders.

In the context of the Himalayan region, the public health and public order containment measures undertaken by states evolved and were like measures taken by states in other parts of the world (Bhaduri, 2021). As previously mentioned, these included mask mandates and contact tracing, lockdowns, curfews, internal mobility restrictions, international border closures, and quarantines. It is important to note that the Himalayan region comprises lower-middle-income and middle-income countries, which presents a different calculation regarding the viability of long-term lockdowns and movement restrictions (Channel News Asia, 2021). Wealthy states have advanced welfare systems (and wealth redistributive mechanisms) to ensure citizens do not fall into poverty, but developing states do not. Thus, states in the Indo-Pacific, including those in the Himalayan region, have a) limited social safety nets and b) large subsistence-wage earning populations who are heavily reliant on the informal sector. The analysis in the remainder of this section assesses the trajectory of response to the COVID-19 pandemic in Nepal, Bhutan and Ladakh, not including vaccination strategies.

4.3.1 Nepal

Nepal's initial efforts to contain the COVID-19 pandemic included efforts undertaken by the public health system to address the pandemic itself – testing and ancillary public order measures such as quarantines, lockdowns, and travel restrictions. The impact of public order responses will be explored in more depth in the final section of the chapter. Nepal's response was led by its Deputy Prime Minister Ishwar Pokrelra, whom the President directed to form a COVID-19 steering committee tasked with addressing the public health and public orders aspect of the COVID-19 pandemic (Pun et al., 2020). Like elsewhere, the pandemic seriously taxed the country's nascent medical capacity, which necessitated rapid and robust changes to the country's fledgling public health system. Between March and May of 2020, the Ministry of Health established isolation wards, set up makeshift hospitals and quarantine centres nationwide and attempted to procure more respiratory ventilation equipment (Pun et al., 2020). In addition, in March of 2020, the Ministry of Health added 1000 hospital beds and 115 ICU spaces in the Kathmandu Valley alone. From mid-2020 onwards, Nepal's public health capacity mirrored other states in the region in terms of treating hospitalized patients. Thus, during this period, the public health system faced concurrent limitations in its ability to a) treat patients (limited isolation wards and ventilation equipment) and b) increase testing capacity. From late January and mid-March 2020, all tests in-country were sent to a laboratory in Hong Kong (UNOCHA, 2021). For example, starting in mid-March of 2020, there was only one functioning laboratory capable of testing COVID-19 in the whole country, and by mid-2020, the Ministry of Health established a network of COVID-19 testing laboratories nationwide (UNOCHA, 2021). As previously noted, the surge of cases in the spring of 2021 brought Nepal's public health system to a point of collapse (Shrestha, 2021). In addition to lack of dedicated ICU wards and ventilation equipment this wave saw a lack of oxygen canisters, which stretched Nepal's already taxed limited public health system (Shrestha, 2021).

Nepal's public order containment measures included a mix of travel restrictions, border closures and domestic lockdowns. Between mid-Jan and mid-May 2020, various inbound travel restrictions were imposed. These included the temporary closure of the China Rasuwagadhi crossing, which brought China–Nepal trade to a standstill, the closure of land borders to third-country nationals, the cancellation of trekking permits, and the suspension of its visa-on-arrival facility (Nagarik Network, 2020). The closure of the land border, particularly in the south of the country, became an important containment tool, as most cases were coming from India as the crisis worsened there (Nagarik Network, 2020). In addition to the international travel restrictions, a national lockdown came into effect on 24 March and ended on 21 July 2020. During this period, school, university, and civil service exams were postponed, and all non-essential government services, including the activities of the country's supreme court and parliament, were postponed (Kathmandu Post, 2021).

4.3.2 Bhutan

Like Nepal, Bhutan's response included public health measures undertaken to treat those stricken with the virus and public order measures to contain its spread. While Bhutan's response was long-term, it had two key phases, the initial outbreak, which did not see a high infection rate, and then a surge in cases following the India-cantered Delta wave in early 2021 (Reuters, 2021). To the extent that Bhutan had a containment strategy, it would be best described as falling into the "zero COVID-19" category. Given Bhutan's small population, low infection rates, and zero community transmission, the state acted aggressively to stop even the smallest outbreaks in 2020 to 2021. (Kaul, 2021).

From the outset, the public health aspects of Bhutan's response were complicated by the general lack of capacity in Bhutan's public health system combined with the country's mountainous and large rural poor population. The lack of capacity in Bhutan's public health system was ameliorated to some degree by an efficient health bureaucracy. In April 2020, within two weeks of the first case, Bhutan's Ministry of Health, under the guidance of the King, quickly endeavoured to increase the state's public health capacity in respect to both treating COVID-19 patients and establishing a local COVID-19 testing regime. For example, after the first cases were detected and the virus spread outside the capital region, the Health Ministry deployed rapid mobile health teams to remote areas (Bhutan Broadcasting Service, 2020a and 2020b). Moreover, in the Mongar District in the country's east, the Ministry of Health converted a royal guest house into a field hospital. It also established a COVID-19 testing facility at Mongar Regional Hospital. Starting in late-April 2020, the Ministry increased testing capacity in the Sarpang and Samste districts, which borders the Indian states of Assam and West Bengal, in response to rising infection rates on the Indian side of the border (Bhutan Broadcasting Service, 2020a and 2020b). Capacity issues in the public health sector were also addressed by foreign assistance, notably from South Korea, which donated US$400,000 for COVID-19 testing capacity, and the World Bank, which fast tracked US$5 million for health infrastructure (Bhutan Broadcasting Service, 2020; Xinhua News Agency, 2021).

Public order responses included border closures, mandatory quarantine for incoming travellers, and intermittent lockdowns between the onset of the pandemic and the worst of the Delta Wave in mid-2021 (Choden, 2021). In the first instance, on 22 March 2020, all land borders with India were closed to foreign and third-country nationals (Choden, 2021). Given Bhutan's porous borders and large numbers of Bhutanese living on the Indian side of the border, measures were taken to evacuate vulnerable communities (Choden, 2021). Specifically, approximately 5000 Bhutanese nationals living in Jaigon in West Bengal were evacuated to Phuntsholing on the Bhutanese side of the border (Bhutan Broadcasting Service, 2020). On 22 March, Druk Air (the country's only airline) stopped flying except for select repatriation flights, which resumed in May 2020 (Bhutan Broadcasting Service, 2020). Interestingly, after the first wave, Bhutan's intermittent internal lockdowns were not followed by further border closures.

Given Bhutan's example as a regional success story in handling the COVID-19 crisis (in respect to low infection rates and the absence of community transmission), there has been a small but growing body of scholarship querying the elements of Bhutan's success. This literature focuses on several areas, including Bhutan's small size and relative isolation, the resiliency and cohesiveness of the Bhutanese population, and their collective confidence in its leadership. For example, Drexler (2021a) highlights the role of Bhutan's 1) investment in disaster and emergency preparedness, 2) its strong emphasis on public health infrastructure (including community-based primary care), and 3) the state's ability to identify and leverage strengths. Tshering and Nima (2021) focus more specifically on the role of leadership in the state's management of the crisis, and argue that Bhutan's success in navigating the crisis can be attributed to leadership style of the King of Bhutan (H.E. Jiyme Wngchuk) and the trust the Bhutanese people have in their leadership. For example, on 22 March 2020, he addressed the nation, telling citizens, "As a small country with a small population, we can overcome any challenge we are faced with if the people and the government work together (Drexler, 2021a and 2021b)." On balance, all these factors likely mitigated worst-case scenarios. While Bhutan's geographic isolation might have played a role in limiting high infection and transmission rates, the strength of Bhutan's public health system and public trust in government cannot be discounted. These factors were all evident in Bhutan's vaccine rollout, which will be discussed in the next section.

4.3.3   Ladakh

The COVID-19 containment measures in Ladakh mirror the measures undertaken by the Indian government in other Himalayan territories and elsewhere in the Himalayan region. Public health measures included the establishment of local testing regimes and increasing Ladakh's limited hospital capacity to treat seriously ill patients (Haji, 2020). Capacity-building measures included oxygen canisters supplied by the World Health Organization and respiratory equipment supplied by the Indian Federal Government (Rehman et al., 2020). In addition, a three-member WHO rapid response team visited the region and advised Ladakhi health officials on best practices regarding respiratory health. Public-order responses included stringent quarantine requirements, border closure, and internal movement restrictions (Rehman et al., 2020). After an initial lockdown period (starting on 22 March 2020) into the spring of 2020, the union territory government adopted an open strategy to boost tourism. In the wake of the Omicron variant, the government reimposed movement restrictions and cancelled all tourism activities in the territory for the winter of 2022.

Several local media outlets reported that in the early stages of the lockdown, the territory government (based in Leh) had difficulty enforcing lockdowns in remote areas, and it took time for officials at the district level to implement and enforce movement control orders (Majid, 2020). Notwithstanding this issue, it was widely reported that in the first wave of the pandemic the deployment of Ladakh's containment measures compared very favourably with measures taken in other union territories, notably Kashmir. Despite effective containment policies in the first wave of the pandemic, high transmission rates in late 2021 have been attributed to reduced testing capacity, superspreader events, and a general reduction in community vigilance.

The analysis in this section highlighted states' response in the Himalayan region to the COVID-19 pandemic. To this end, we see that states in the region present similar but different internal dynamics regarding the spread of the virus, and all undertook similar measures that reflected standard operating procedures (SOPs). All states faced a low level in terms of public health capacity, and none of the territories discussed had any indigenous testing capacity. Narratives on responses to the pandemic vary across the states. Bhutan has been lauded as a success story; Ladakh has performed favourably compared to other Indian union territories; and Nepal's response has been judged less favourably.

4.4   Part 3: Vaccination Strategies

The rapid development of effective vaccines has without question been the most critical innovation in the containment of the pandemic since its outset. Notwithstanding the critique that vaccines did not "deliver" on the assurance that they would stop transmission and facilitate a return to normal, it is widely accepted that vaccination has dramatically reduced death and hospitalization rates, especially amongst vulnerable groups. Given the time scale and complexity of the situation, the initial tranche of vaccines came from states with capacity in this area. In the first instance, vaccines were developed by Western consortiums (USA, Germany, UK, and Sweden), China, and Russia. From early on (mid-2020) in the pandemic, China used "vaccine diplomacy" to extend its national interests, both in the Indo-Pacific and further afield. To the extent that Western-produced vaccines were acknowledged as being more efficacious, they were slower to market, despite the swift development of vaccines production and distribution delays and then political wrangling over export shoring up domestic supply before exporting stock (Oehler & Vega, 2021). Indeed, as previously noted, for states in the Global South, the major issues associated with the development and execution of the COVID-19 vaccination strategy relate to deeper issues associated with the sources and distribution.

Procurement strategies balanced access and speed against efficacy for states in the Global South. While Chinese and Russian vaccines were fast to market, they were objectively less effective and debatably were developed with less rigorous testing and approval processes (Chalwe, 2021). On the other hand, access to Western vaccines also proved challenging. While more efficacious (especially the mRNA vaccines), the distribution of these vaccines got mired in production and distribution delays and domestic politics, which demanded export restrictions. Thus, wealthy states who did not produce vaccines used their resources and influence to secure large quantities of "A-grade vaccines" at the expense of states in the Global South (Mirza & Rauhala, 2021). Despite supposed multi-lateral solutions such as the WHO's COVAX program, vaccine diplomacy devolved into a version of realpolitik (Fidler, 2021).

Vaccination rates, as well as procurement and distribution policies, have varied within the Himalayan region. Bhutan has the highest vaccination rates, with 74.2% of the population fully vaccinated, 100% receiving the first dose (Schiffling & Phelan, 2021). Interestingly, Bhutan could deploy its vaccine regime quickly to the extent that 93% of adults received the first dose within two weeks. Nepal achieved an overall vaccination rate of 63.9%. Moreover, Ladakh achieved a vaccination rate of 50% of the adult population (100% having received first doses). The dynamics associated with vaccine procurement and roll-outs correlate with broader structural trends highlighted in the section. Bhutan has the highest vaccination rate and has the smallest population and most functioning health system. As a union territory of India, Ladakh does not maintain its vaccination procurement agendas; instead, its vaccination distribution is bound up in India's national strategy. Moreover, Nepal, for its part, has the disadvantage of being large and having the least integrated or functional public health system in the Himalayan region, which has impacted distribution (UNOCHA, 2021). Regional geopolitics have also figured into vaccine procurement strategies, particularly in Nepal and Bhutan. Bhutan has relied exclusively on Western-developed vaccines, while Nepal has relied on a mix of Indian-produced AstraZeneca via the Serum Institute of India (SII) and Chinese-produced Sinopharm vaccines.

The remainder of this section will analyse the country-level dynamics associated with vaccination rates, procurement policy, and distribution strategy in Nepal, Bhutan, and Ladakh.

4.4.1 Nepal

As previously mentioned, as of February 2022, Nepal had achieved an overall vaccination rate of 63.9% and administered 36,576,224 doses of vaccines via nine approved vaccines (Reuters, 2021). Initially, the UK-developed AstraZeneca was supposed to be the mainstay of Nepal's procurement strategy from a combination of sources, including bilateral procurement via the government of India via the COVAX program (Reuters 2021). In February 2021, the Indian government gave Nepal 1 million does as a grant, and with another 2 million doses purchased from the SII (Reuters, 2021). The first 1 million doses arrived in the country on 21 February, while the remaining doses were delayed due to production delays and an Indian-imposed export ban. The delays from the SII and the slowness of the COVAX program resulted in the diversification of supply to include use of the Chinese-developed Sinopharm, which played an essential role in meeting demand in the first half of 2021. In the summer of 2021, the supply of vaccines increased steadily with the arrival of a further 8 million doses of Sinopharm and 1.5 million doses of single-jab Jansen/Johnson & Johnson vaccine, which was granted to the government of Nepal by the USA via the COVAX program. Notably, this included approximately 800,000 doses, which arrived on 29 March.

Nepal's vaccine program was formally launched on 27 January and expanded significantly in the second half of 2021, passing the 50% ratio in December 2021 (Al Jazeera, 2021). Like elsewhere, the state experienced significant issues related to the supply and distribution of vaccines. For example, in June of 2021, Nepal had fully vaccinated a total of 2.4% of its population, while the UK vaccinated 45% (Callamard, 2021). In the first phase (January-March 2021) 434,000 doses were administered, with eligibility reserved for frontline workers/health workers, elderly people (living in care homes), supporting staffers at health facilities, female community health volunteers, prisoners, and security personnel, (Kathmandu Post, 2021). The vaccine used in this phase came from AstraZeneca produced by SII. In the second phase of the program (March–May 2021), 1.3 million vaccine doses were administered, with eligibility expanded to include those over 65 and persons working in the service and transport sectors. This phase was carried out in two sub-phases that used the SII AstraZeneca and then, following the Indian-imposed export ban, Sinopharm.

Despite the overall efficacy of Nepal's vaccine program, particularly from the second half of 2021 onwards, core weaknesses in the public health system impacted the roll-out of the vaccination program. Like other states, Nepal has had issues with the management of its vaccination system in respect to registration processes, tracking vaccination status, staging, scheduling of vaccination appointments, and communicating vaccination locations and eligibility guidelines for the second doses (Callamard, 2021). These deficiencies were amplified by the fact that the "scaling-up" of Nepal's vaccination program (in May–July 2021) coincided with the worst of the South Asian wave of the pandemic, which devastated an already strained public health system (Callamard, 2021).

4.4.2 Bhutan

Despite its small size and limited capacity, Bhutan's vaccination program has achieved impressive results by regional and global standards. As previously noted, as of February 2022, it had achieved an overall vaccination rate of 74.2%. The country's vaccine procurement strategy relied almost exclusively on Western-developed vaccines, notable AstraZeneca and Moderna (Xinhua News Agency, 2021). Between January and March 2021, Bhutan received 550,000 doses of Astra-Zeneca from India, which included an initial delivery of 150,000 doses in January and an additional 400,000 doses in March (Royal Government of Bhutan, 2022). In July 2021, it received an aggregate of 900,000 additional doses, including 500,000 doses of Moderna from the USA, approximately 400,000 doses of AstraZeneca from several European countries, and a small consignment (50,000 doses) of Sinopharm from China (Royal Government of Bhutan, 2022).

Bhutan's vaccination program was launched on 27 March 2021 and was delivered in two phases. The first phase was implemented in one week, whereby 05% of Bhutan's population secured first doses on AstraZeneca in a seven-day period (Schiffling & Phelan, 2021). The second phase was rolled out in July 2021 following additional doses as described above. Phases 1 and 2 administered a total of 1.51 million doses (Schiffling & Phelan, 2021).

Several factors facilitated the swiftness and success of Bhutan's vaccination program. First, the state was able to procure enough doses of vaccine to administer first doses to the country's entire adult population (Whitecross, 2021). Second, Bhutan's strategic relationship with India allowed it to bypass India's export controls (Bhonsale, 2020). Third, public health authorities successfully leveraged synergies in the country's effective community-based care clinics as distribution points for vaccine delivery while putting the country's well-developed helicopter rescue service to work delivering vaccines to remote communities (Whitecross, 2021). Fourth, the roll-out of the second phase was "functional" due to the availably of vaccines and because, unlike Nepal, Bhutan's public health system was not encumbered with a catastrophic outbreak at the time (Drexler, 2020).

4.4.3 Ladakh

As a union territory of India, decisions regarding the procurement and distribution of vaccines lie with the central government in New Delhi. According to official sources, the federal government of India allocates vaccine supplies to states and union territories on the basis of population and infection rates (Dutta, 2021; Economic Times of India, 2021). In this sense, Ladakh had an advantage to the extent that it was part of India's state distribution network and received locally developed and manufactured AstraZeneca (Dutta, 2021). Furthermore, as we highlighted earlier, by Indian national standards, Ladakh's identification and containment measures compare very favourably to other union territories (i.e., Kashmir).

Ladakh's program began on 16 April 2021 and achieved a 100% first-dose vaccination rate by early July (Administration of Union Territory of Ladakh, 2021). In the first phase, 89,404 people received first doses, focusing on the two largest districts in the country, Leh and Kargil (Administration of Union Territory of Ladakh, 2021). This phase included the elderly and 18- to 44-year-olds working in the hospitality sector. The second phase administered second doses to 60,936 people (Administration of Union Territory of Ladakh, 2021). There were reports of some discrepancy in the provision of second doses. The Leh district has a fully vaccinated rate of 58%, while the more remote Kargil and remote areas have lower second-dose rates of 42% (Economic Times of India, 2021. Rather than issues associated with local distribution capacity and or vaccine hesitancy, the slowness in achieving a higher second dose rate lies with the overall availability of the vaccine and the extent to which the central government controls the supply depending on need elsewhere in the country (Economic Times of India, 2021.

This section has examined the strategies and policies undertaken to procure and then distribute vaccines. Several trends emerge from the analysis. First, all states in the Himalayan region have benefitted from India's production capacity and it's "neighbourhood first" approach in vaccine diplomacy and were able to deploy vaccination programs quickly using Indian-manufactured vaccines. Second, there was a subtle geo-political note to vaccine procurement strategies, with all states relying heavily (in the first instance) on Indian or Western-developed vaccines. And two of the three territories discussed (Ladakh and Bhutan) were not subject to Indian-imposed export controls. Third, while all states developed vaccination strategies and achieved average or higher than average rates of vaccination, the efficacy of the strategies was impacted greatly by realities on the ground. Bhutan's program has been objectively more effective than Nepal's, in terms of the procurement and distribution, which reflects the speed with which it was able to secure vaccines and the efficacy of its public health system.

4.5 Part 4: Non-Traditional Security and the Impact of the COVID-19 Pandemic

So far, this chapter has examined responses to the COVID-19 pandemic undertaken by states in terms of public health, public order, and vaccination strategies. The analysis reveals that infection and death rates (particularly in Bhutan and Ladakh) were lower than average by regional standards. Dynamics associated with the COVID-19 pandemic in the Himalayas show a corollary relationship between state capacity and better/worse outcomes. Furthermore, death and infection rates (particularly in Bhutan and Ladakh) were lower than average by regional standards. In the case of Bhutan, an effective vaccine procurement strategy, a robust community health system, high levels of public trust in the state, and effective policy communication all comingled to create comparatively better outcomes.

Notwithstanding the Himalayan region's comparatively successful handling of the COVID-19 pandemic, its impact on communities at the intra-state level should not be ignored. In this sense, the COVID-19 pandemic provides us with a case study of not only how a region has dealt with an enormous public health crisis but also the complex inter-relationship between the supposed spheres of NTS. As previously discussed, NTS is understood as security threats and challenges a) that are trans-national in scope and b) whose resolution do not primarily involve the application of force (Anthony et al., 2017). Analysed at sectoral levels, the spheres of non-traditional security include economy, food, migration, health, societal security, and gender. At the same time, the COVID-19 pandemic can be understood within the context of "health security," i.e., as a once-in-a-century public health crisis marked by the collapse of public health infrastructure and catastrophic loss of life. At the same time, we can also observe the knock-on effects of the pandemic in terms of how state responses have set off multiple concurrent crises in other NTS spheres. Most significantly, beyond the health crisis itself, the pandemic's impact was felt in economic contraction, and travel and movement restrictions (Channel News Asia, 2021; First Post, 2020). These have raised levels of insecurity across multiple spheres of NTS spheres that will be felt in most societies for decades to come.

While the impact of the pandemic has been uneven across the Himalayan region, all states have experienced significant and far-reaching disruption driven by the synergistic effects of the pandemic on one hand and state responses to contain outbreaks on the other. Economic contraction resulted in higher unemployment, which pushed already marginal communities into poverty (First Post, 2020). At the same time, state-imposed movement restrictions resulted in food insecurity. The combined effect of economic and food insecurity in some states, notably Nepal, has impacted social cohesion and exacerbated inter-communal tensions, while the Indian Himalayan region has by all accounts experienced heightened pandemic-related structural gender-based power inequity ("COVID-19 in the Himalaya", 2021). The remainder of this section will examine the impact on the spheres of NTS regarding economic insecurity, food insecurity, and societal security.

4.5.1 Economic Security

Within the context of NTS, *economic security* is defined broadly as the ability of countries to follow their choice of policies to develop the national economy in the manner desired (Anthony et al., 2017). To the extent that all states in the Global South experience economic security challenges, the dynamics associated with the pandemic have significantly impacted the capacity of states to deliver economic security. In this sense, economic insecurity in the form of resource scarcity is experienced equally by states who lack the resources to "deliver" or manage economic policy and by residents who deal with the day-to-day to consequences of poverty. For our purposes, economic insecurity associated with the COVID-19 pandemic in the Himalayan region manifested itself in several ways, including contractions within the region's tourism sector, losses in overseas remittances from Himalayan overseas workers, and the contraction which impacted the region's informal sector, which accounts for 40–50% of the region's economies (World Vision, 2021). In macro terms, economies in the South Asian region contracted by 7.7% in FY2020, with GDP reductions of –6.8% and –2.1% growth respectively in Bhutan Nepal (The World Bank, 2020; The World Trade Organization, 2021). Moreover, rising levels of economic insecurity exacerbate worse outcomes in other NTS spheres, such as rising levels of food insecurity and worsening social cohesion.

In the case of Nepal, pandemic-driven economic insecurity had multiple drivers. In the first instance, travel and movement restrictions decimated the county's tourism sector, which employs large numbers of Nepalese both formally and informally and is a vital source of foreign currency. The pandemic also exacerbated structural dynamics in Nepal's economy, specifically the state's reliance on foreign worker remittances to fund its budget (26% of GDP) and a substantial informal sector that employs approximately 50% of the workforce and many women (The World Trade Organization, 2021). Thus, pandemic-related restrictions resulted in a contraction in overseas remittances and saw many women in the informal section completely jobless. A report published by the Asia Foundation in (2021) found that in mid-2020, 1 in 10 Nepalese were jobless while 3 in 10 had suffered some income loss. Where Nepalese employed in the formal sector typically suffered wage reductions, people employed in the informal sector were often left completely jobless (The Asia Foundation, 2021). According to a World Vision (2021) survey, at the height of the pandemic, average incomes amongst respondents went from $130 to $43 per month, and 86% took loans, mostly from informal lenders.

While pandemic-driven economic precarity in Nepal was particularly acute, the trends discussed above mirrored the Himalayan region to a large degree. In the cases of Ladakh and Bhutan, while both are smaller and objectively "less poor," they are also economically almost entirely reliant tourism and trekking. Thus, the ongoing cancellation of the trekking activities continues to have a dire impact on rural economies in Bhutan and Lakh.

4.5.1.1   Food Security

According to the United Nations, food security is defined in such a way that all people, at all times, have physical, social, and economic access to sufficient, safe, and nutritious food that meets their food preferences and dietary needs for an active and healthy life (IFPRI, 2023). The UN Food and Agriculture Program (FAO) elaborates several dimensions of food security, including food availability, food access, utilization, and stability (FAO, 2006). Where food availability and stability are structural and managed by states, utilization and stability often vary within states by location and socio-economic status. Himalayan states, particularly Ladakh and Bhutan, are geographically remote, high in altitude with limited capacity of arable farming land. States in this region meet their food security needs through a mix of local farming and imports from India and China. It should be noted that states in this region are semi-food insecure at the best of times. Lower-middle-income states have limited capacity to ameliorate food insecurity using economic statecraft.

In the Himalayan region, the COVID-19 pandemic brought on a multidimensional food security crisis with concurrent impacts on food availability, food access, utilization, and stability. Overall, the region's rate of severe food insecurity rose dramatically from 19% in the pre-pandemic period to 35% at the height of the pandemic (World Vision, 2021). The closure of borders made it more difficult for states to secure food availability via the usual import mechanisms, while internal movement restrictions impacted states' ability to distribute foodstuffs nationally. Economic insecurity greatly impacted food access (i.e., reduced wages and joblessness), which meant that people could not afford to buy the food available, resulting in price inflation. Food utilization was impacted to the extent that pandemic conditions curtailed the availability of certain foods (imports) and made it more difficult for the state to help existing food insecure communities. Moreover, food stability was also affected to the extent that pandemic conditions brought on crises of availability and access. Thus, to varying degrees, these factors made difficult for states to ensure supply stability.

Furthermore, data from Nepal gives some insight into the depth of the pandemic-driven food insecurity and the relationship between economic and food security. For example, the previously mentioned World Vision survey conducted at the height of the pandemic found that 87% of respondents noted that prices on essential goods had gone up, 72% did not have access to recommended food diversity, and 26% did not have access to agricultural outputs (World Vision, 2021). The survey also showed a dramatic shift in the focus of household spending. During the height of the pandemic, an average of 46% was allocated to food (World Vision, 2021). This survey also shows a distinctly gendered aspect to food insecurity to the extent that female-headed households were on average more food insecure than male-headed households (World Vision, 2021).

4.5.2 Societal Security and Social Cohesion

The concept of societal security evolved from the Copenhagen School of Security Studies and focused on the ability of a society to persist in its essential character (Anthony et al., 2017). And within this context, social cohesion plays an essential role in the state's ability to maintain societal security. Conceptually, social cohesion can be understood vertically and horizontally – vertically as the relationship between people and government and horizontally among various social groups in society (ethnic and religious). Factors such as wars, mass migration, and sudden and catastrophic changes to public life brought on by events such as pandemics and natural disasters can all challenge societal security and, with it, social cohesion. Dynamics associated with the pandemic have presented both horizontal and vertical challenges to societal security. For example, in many Western states, responses to the pandemic have eroded vertical social cohesion in terms of public support for, and trust in, government, and horizontal social cohesion has exacerbated political divisions and inter-communal conflict. The pandemic has increased horizontal tensions in several contexts and states. In North America, there has been a marked rise in anti-Asian (specifically anti-Chinese) sentiment, reflecting a reactionary right-wing trope that the "Chinese" were to blame for the pandemic. In addition, the politicization of mask mandates and movement restrictions has unfolded around partisan life and deepened divisions.

By regional and global standards, states within the Himalayan region have high levels of societal security and vertical social cohesion. By all accounts, pandemic conditions have done little to change this reality. Despite the success in maintaining vertical social cohesion, many horizontal challenges exist, which are largely an extension of pandemic-driven economic insecurity. A United Nations Development Programme (UNDP) report (2021) highlights, at a Himalayan sub-region level, three pandemic-related contexts which challenge social cohesion, which include 1) returning labour migrants, 2) suspicion and fear of ethno-religious minority groups, and 3) discrimination stemming from social distancing:

1 As previously mentioned, Nepal had to resettle many jobless returning labour migrants who lost overseas jobs across Asia-Pacific and Middle East and North Africa (MENA) regions. The increased economic competition among recently returned job-seeking migrants and the practical difficulties of reintegration, such as housing for returning migrants without family support and short-term livelihood support, presented a challenge to the reintegration of the returning migrants.

2 Resource scarcity often exacerbates inter-group tensions. In the Himalayan context, these tensions can be seen in ethno-religious groups and inter-caste interactions. For example, in Bhutan, ongoing tensions between the majority Buddhist Ngalop and minority Hindu Lhotshampa communities highlight the issues associated with access to resources. In this case, the Lhotshampa community feels that state responses regarding pandemic-related economic support have not been given equally

3 In Nepal, various civil society experts have warned that masking and social distancing might increase caste-based discrimination to the extent that these regulations marginalize already marginalized communities.

In addition to these, the other context through which we can view the social cohesion issue is the impact on vulnerable and disadvantaged groups who are not ethno-religious minorities. Beyond the marginalization associated with ethno-religion minority status, this can also be examined in the context of patriarchy and the impact of the COVID-19 pandemic on gender-based outcomes. Dynamics associated with the pandemic made life appreciably worse for the vulnerable. As previously discussed, women experienced worse poor food and economic security outcomes. This fact was substantiated in a report published by the Asia Foundation (2021), which noted that Nepali women work in the informal sector in greater numbers than men and suffer more economic impact than men working in the formal sector. The former being more reliant on the informal sector and more likely to face pandemic-related joblessness.

This section has proffered a conceptual linkage between the COVID-19 pandemic and NTS It has examined how pandemic conditions in the Himalayan region have challenged spheres of NTS and the extent to which economic contraction, border closures, and movement restrictions have impacted economic and food security outcomes and social cohesion. It also demonstrated the interconnection between economic, food, and societal NTS spheres and the challenges of state response therein. It also showed that security outcomes were inexorably worse for already vulnerable communities, particularly in Nepal.

4.6 Conclusion

This chapter has offered a preliminary analysis of the COVID-19 pandemic in the Himalayan region. The first section examined the scale of the outbreak. It argued that, to the extent that the COVID-19 pandemic ravaged South Asia, its impact on the Himalayan region was less severe, at least in relative terms. It also argued that while states in the region faced similar challenges, there were also differences. Nepal is substantially more "globalized" than either Ladakh or Bhutan and had to re-integrate a large number of jobless returning labour migrants. The second section examined the response regarding containment measures and found that all states undertook similar measures and implemented border closures and movement restrictions. The third section examined the vaccination strategies and found that all states relied on bilateral relationships with India to shore up vaccine supplies. Bhutan's vaccination was effective due to its health system and its ability to secure vaccines. The final section examined the pandemic's impact in terms of NTS and how it challenged economic, food, and societal security.

While more data needs to be collected at the country and community levels, the three-country comparison presented in the chapter shows several trends. First, there seems to be a correlation between state capacity and the overall effectiveness of state responses in the Himalayan region. In this sense, Bhutan emerges as the overall "winner" in handling the crisis, ranging from the initial outbreak to vaccination. While it is not the most developed state in the region, it has an effective public health system and functional health bureaucracy. Bhutan's success has been the subject of considerable discussion. The factors attributed to this success range from the personal attributes of its leadership to the efficacy of its health system, its small size and low population density, and the lack of global connectivity. Notwithstanding Bhutan's objective success in managing the pandemic, there is an important caveat: the lack of Ladakh- and Bhutan-specific data regarding food and economic security outcomes. Second, the success of Bhutan in handling the pandemic shows that vertical social cohesion (i.e., trust in government) matters and results in more compliance. Finally, the COVID-19 pandemic began as a health security crisis that quickly snowballed into multi-dimensional crises encompassing multiple spheres of NTS. This reality shows the impact of NTS challenges and the complex inter-relationship between spheres of NTS health security, economic security, and food security.

It is important to note that "the history" of the pandemic, including its impact on the Himalayan region, is still being written as it unfolds. As such, this chapter has been intended as a provisional discussion of the scale of the impact and how states have managed their responses and its impact. Clearly there is need for more analysis on various aspects of the pandemic's impact and way in which states in the region have responded. We see that overall numbers were, by regional and global standards, low, which can be understood in terms of low population and density and better than average state responses.

Notes

1 The opinions expressed in this work are those of the author and do not reflect the views of the National Defense College or the United Arab Emirates government.
2 The Hindu Kush Himalayan (HKH) region includes Afghanistan, Bangladesh, Bhutan, China, India, Myanmar Nepal, and Pakistan.

Bibliography

Administration of Union Territory of Ladakh. (2021). *Covid-19: Ladakh achieves 100% vaccination with first dose*. Retrieved from https://ladakh.nic.in/covid-19-ladakh-achieves-100-vaccination-with-first-dose/

Al Jazeera. (2021). Nepal to vaccinate all adults by mid-April: Health minister. Retrieved November 24, 2021, from https://www.aljazeera.com/news/2021/11/11/nepal-covid-vaccination-adults-mid-april-health-minister

Anthony, M., Emmers, R., & Acharya, A. (2017). *Non-traditional security in Asia*. Sage.

Aroor, S. (2021). India gripped by Covid, China quietly hardens positions in depth areas of Ladakh. *India Today*. Retrieved November 24, 2021, from https://www.indiatoday.in/amp/india/story/india-gripped-by-covid-china-quietly-hardens-positions-in-depth-areas-of-ladakh-1796760-2021-04-30

Australian Himalayan Foundation. (2021). COVID-19 in the Himalaya. Retrieved November 24, 2021, from https://www.australianhimalayanfoundation.org.au/covid-19/

Bahukhandi, K., Agarwal, S., & Singhal, S. (2020). Impact of lockdown Covid-19 pandemic on Himalayan environment. *International Journal of Environmental Analytical Chemistry*, 1–15.

Bhaduri, S. (2021). Comparing COVID-19 pandemic responses of three South Asian countries-Bhutan, Sri Lanka, and Bangladesh. *The Indian Practitioner*, *73*(11), 7–14. Retrieved November 25, 2021, from https://www.semanticscholar.org/paper/Impact-of-lockdown-Covid-19-pandemic-on-himalayan-Bahukhandi-Agarwal/4bd70176f7cdc03cb0ebd5ed644b699774c98ff0

Bhonsale, M. (2020). Bhutan: Covid-19 cooperation push to India relations. Observer Research Foundation. Retrieved from https://www.orfonline.org/research/south-asia-weekly-report-volume-xiii-45/

Bhutan Broadcasting Service. (2020a). Bhutanese evacuees from Jaigaon well looked after by the Office of the Gyalpoi Zimpon. Retrieved March 7, 2022, from https://web.archive.org/web/20200414092542/http://www.bbs.bt/news/?p=130765

Bhutan Broadcasting Service. (2020b). Republic of Korea provides a grant support of USD 400,000 to Bhutan. Retrieved March 7, 2022, from https://web.archive.org/web/20200603032807/http://www.bbs.bt/news/?p=132641

Callamard, A. (2021). Covid vaccine in short supply in Nepal: A week to help pull nation back from the brink – What Britain must do. Amnesty International. Retrieved from https://www.amnesty.org/en/latest/news/2021/06/covid-vaccine-in-short-supply-in-nepal-a-week-to-help-pull-nation-back-from-the-brink-what-britain-must-do/

Centers for Disease Control and Prevention. (2022). *Similarities and differences between Flu and COVID-19*. Retrieved March 7, 2022, from https://www.cdc.gov/flu/symptoms/flu-vs-covid19.htm

Chalise, H. (2020). COVID-19 situation and challenges for Nepal. *Asia Pacific Journal of Public Health*, *32*(5), 281–282. https://doi.org/10.1177/1010539520932709

Chalwe, M. (2021). Vaccine inequality: If not for China, would the West even be tackling it? *South China Morning Post*. Retrieved March 7, 2022, from https://www.scmp.com/comment/opinion/article/3142138/vaccine-inequality-if-not-china-would-west-even-be-tackling-it

Channel News Asia. (2021). Death in the Himalayas: Poverty, fear, stretched resources propel India's COVID-19 crisis. Retrieved November 24, 2021, from https://www.channelnewsasia.com/asia/death-himalayas-poverty-fear-stretched-resources-propel-indias-covid-19-crisis-1408996

Choden, K. (2021). An overview of Bhutan's recovery efforts. Friedrich Neumann Foundation. Retrieved from https://www.freiheit.org/south-asia/overview-bhutans-recovery-efforts

Dialogue Earth. (2021). Latest Covid-19 wave engulfs unprepared Himalayas. [Blog]. Retrieved November 24, 2021, from https://www.thethirdpole.net/en/livelihoods/covid-19-engulfs-unprepared-himalayas/

Drexler, K. (2020). Government extension, agroecology, and sustainable food systems in Belize milpa farming communities: A socio-ecological systems approach. *Journal of Agriculture, Food Systems, and Community Development*, *9*(3), 85–97. https://doi.org/10.5304/jafscd.2020.093.001

Drexler, M. (2021a). How Bhutan has kept COVID-19 at bay. T.H Chan School of Public Health, Harvard University. Retrieved November 24, 2021, from https://www.hsph.harvard.edu/news/hsph-in-the-news/how-bhutan-has-kept-covid-19-at-bay/

Drexler, M. (2021b). The unlikeliest Pandemic success story. *The Atlantic*. Retrieved November 24, 2021, from https://www.theatlantic.com/international/archive/2021/02/coronavirus-pandemic-bhutan/617976/

Dutta, S. (2021). Ladakh first Union Territory to achieve 100% Covid vaccination with first dose. *The Times of India*. Retrieved March 7, 2022, from https://timesofindia.indiatimes.com/city/srinagar/ladakh-first-union-territory-to-achieve-100-covid-vaccination-with-first-dose/articleshow/84298625.cms

Economic Times of India. (2021). COVID-19 vaccine distribution among states done in transparent manner: Centre. Retrieved February 26, 2022, from https://economictimes.

indiatimes.com/news/india/covid-19-vaccine-distribution-among-states-done-in-transparent-manner-centre/articleshow/83807438.cms?from=mdr.

Fidler, D. (2021). Global Health's reckoning with realpolitik. Council on Foreign Relations. Retrieved from https://www.thinkglobalhealth.org/article/global-healths-reckoning-realpolitik

First Post. (2020). COVID-19 crisis highlights long-term neglect of Himalayan women in determining water policies. Retrieved November 24, 2021, from https://www.firstpost.com/long-reads/covid-19-crisis-highlights-long-term-neglect-of-himalayan-women-marginalised-groups-in-determining-water-policies-8298361.html.

Food and Agriculture Organization of the United Nations. (2006). *The state of food and agriculture: Food aid for food security?* FAO Agriculture Series No. 37. FAO.

Government of Nepal Ministry of Health and Population. (2021). Health sector response to COVID-19. Retrieved from https://covid19.mohp.gov.np/covid/englishSituationReport/6127790a38080_SitRep564_COVID-19_26-08-2021_EN.pdf

Haji, M. (2020). Ladakh is winning the war on COVID-19 but the voices of the people are diminishing. *The Wire*. Retrieved November 24, 2021, from https://thewire.in/government/ladakh-is-winning-the-war-on-covid-19-but-the-voices-of-the-people-are-diminishing

Administrator, How Coronavirus has affected the lives of people at the Himalayas? (2020). [Blog]. Retrieved November 24, 2021, from https://www.moxtain.com/blogs/impact-of-coronavirus-on-himalayan-local

Human Rights Watch. (2021). Nepal: Act to avert looming covid-19 disaster. Retrieved from https://www.hrw.org/news/2021/05/10/nepal-act-avert-looming-covid-19-disaster

ICIMOD. (2020). *COVID-19 impact and policy responses in the Hindu Kush Himalaya.* Retrieved from https://lib.icimod.org/record/34863

Indian Express. (2020). High altitude, high UV rays keep Ladakh's COVID-19 numbers low, say experts. Retrieved November 24, 2021, from https://indianexpress.com/article/india/high-altitude-high-uv-rays-keep-ladakhs-covid-19-numbers-low-say-experts-6527790/.

International Food Policy Research Institute (IFPRI). (2023). *Title of the report* (Report No. 136727). International Food Policy Research Institute. https://ebrary.ifpri.org/utils/getfile/collection/p15738coll2/id/136727/filename/136938.pdf

Kafle, B. (2020). Social cohesion in the context of COVID-19 in Nepal. https://www.np.undp.org/content/nepal/en/home/blog/2020/Social-cohesion-in-the-context-of-COVID19-in-Nepal.html [Blog]. Retrieved March 4, 2022, from https://www.np.undp.org/content/nepal/en/home/blog/2020/Social-cohesion-in-the-context-of-COVID19-in-Nepal.html

Kathmandu Post. (2021). Nepal's vaccination status. Retrieved February 25, 2022, from https://kathmandupost.com/health/2021/05/12/nepal-s-vaccination-status

Kaul, N. (2021). Small state, big example: Covid pandemic management in Bhutan. *Critical Studies on Security*, *9*(1), 58–62. https://doi.org/10.1080/21624887.2021.1904359

Krishna, S. (2021). *Bhutan: A coronavirus success story*. Carnegie India Center. Retrieved from https://carnegieindia.org/2020/05/21/bhutan-coronavirus-success-story-pub-81856

Lse.ac.uk. (2022). COVID-19 eroding youth trust in political leadership and institutions | LSE Research. Retrieved March 7, 2022, from https://www.lse.ac.uk/research/research-for-the-world/politics/the-political-scar-of-epidemics-why-covid-19-is-eroding-young-peoples-trust-in-their-leaders-and-political-institutions

Majid, Z. (2020). Ladakh shows how to deal with corona virus pandemic. *Deccan Herald*. Retrieved March 7, 2022, from https://www.deccanherald.com/national/north-and-central/ladakh-shows-how-to-deal-with-coronavirus-pandemic-821272.htm

Mirza, A., & Rauhala, E. (2021). Here's just how unequal the global coronavirus vaccine rollout has been. *Washington Post*. Retrieved March 7, 2022, from https://www.washingtonpost.com/world/interactive/2021/coronavirus-vaccine-inequality-global/

Mukherjee, S. (2021). Why does the pandemic seem to be hitting some countries harder than others? *The New Yorker*. Retrieved March 15, 2022, from https://www.newyorker.

com/magazine/2021/03/01/why-does-the-pandemic-seem-to-be-hitting-some-countries-harder-than-others

Nagarik Network. (2020). *Nepal-China Rasuwagadhi border point to be sealed for 15 days from Wednesday*. Retrieved March 7, 2022, from https://myrepublica.nagariknetwork.com/news/85919/

Neuman, S. (2021). COVID-19 reaches mount Everest as Nepal Struggles with record Infections. *National Public Radio (NPR)*. Retrieved November 24, 2021, from https://www.npr.org/sections/coronavirus-live-updates/2021/05/05/993837355/covid-19-reaches-mount-everest-as-nepal-struggles-with-record-infections.

Oehler, R., & Vega, V. (2021). Conquering COVID: How global vaccine inequality risks prolonging the pandemic. *Open Forum Infectious Diseases*, *8*(10). https://doi.org/10.1093/ofid/ofab443

Pun, S., Mandal, S., Bhandari, L., Jha, S., Rajbhandari, S., Mishra, A., et al. (2020). Understanding COVID-19 in Nepal. *Journal Of Nepal Health Research Council*, *18*(1), 126–127. https://doi.org/10.33314/jnhrc.v18i1.2629

Ranjit, S., Sigdel, S., Ozaki, A., Kotera, Y., Bhandari, D., Regmi, P., & Rabaan, A. (2020). Impact of COVID-19 on tourism in Nepal. *Journal of Travel Medicine*, *27*(6). Retrieved November 25, 2021, from https://pubmed.ncbi.nlm.nih.gov/32634211/

Rehman, T., Goel, K., Arora, A., Angchuk, P., Samphel, R., Kiran, T., et al. (2020). The successful containment of COVID-19 outbreak in Union Territory of Ladakh, India, 2020. *Journal Of Family Medicine and Primary Care*, *9*(11), 5574. https://doi.org/10.4103/jfmpc.jfmpc_1413_20

Reuters. (2021). COVID-19 Tracker: Bhutan. Retrieved November 24, 2021, from https://graphics.reuters.com/world-coronavirus-tracker-and-maps/countries-and-territories/bhutan/

Royal Government of Bhutan. (2022). *Vaccines for Bhutan*. Retrieved from https://www.gov.bt/covid19/13-07-21-Press-Release-Vac/

Schiffling, S., & Phelan, C. (2021). *What the world can learn from Bhutan's rapid COVID vaccine rollout*. The Conversation. Retrieved from https://theconversation.com/what-the-world-can-learn-from-bhutans-rapid-covid-vaccine-rollout-168341

Schoff, A., Joshi, K., Adhikari, P., & Pant, G. (2020). The effect of the COVID-19 pandemic on mountain communities of the Indian Himalaya. *Mountain Sentinels*. Retrieved November 24, 2021, from https://mountainsentinels.org/the-effect-of-the-covid-19-pandemic-on-mountain-communities-of-the-indian-himalaya/

Shrestha, S. (2021). Nepal says its Covid response is under control – Everyone can see it's not true. *The Guardian*. Retrieved November 24, 2021, from https://www.theguardian.com/global-development/commentisfree/2021/may/11/nepal-says-its-covid-response-is-under-control-everyone-can-see-its-not-true

Syailendrawati, R., Chan, A., Leach-Kemon, K., & Mokdad, A. (2022). *What happens when zero-COVID countries lift restrictions: How Singapore, Australia, Vietnam, and others are transitioning*. Council on Foreign Relation. Retrieved from https://www.thinkglobalhealth.org/article/what-happens-when-zero-covid-countries-lift-restrictions

Tamang, S., & Dorji, T. (2021). Challenges and response to the second major local outbreak of COVID-19 in Bhutan. *Asia Pacific Journal of Public Health*, *33*(8), 953–955. Retrieved November 25, 2021, from https://pubmed.ncbi.nlm.nih.gov/33829879/

The Asia Foundation. (2021). *The impact of the covid-19 pandemic on employment in middle-order cities of Nepal a RAPID ASSESSMENT*. Retrieved from https://asiafoundation.org/wp-content/uploads/2021/04/Impact-of-the-Covid-19-Pandemic-on-Employment-in-Middle-order-Cities-of-Nepal.pdf

The Hindustan Times. (2020). With curbs relaxed, Covid-19 cases spike in Himalayan states. Retrieved November 24, 2021, from https://www.hindustantimes.com/india-news/with-curbs-relaxed-covid-19-cases-spike-in-himalayan-states/story-GZ2yF3rRyqmliwJtyWVk7I_amp.html

The World Bank. (2020). *COVID-19 impact on Nepal's economy hits hardest informal sector*. Retrieved from https://www.worldbank.org/en/news/press-release/2020/10/08/covid-19-impact-on-nepals-economy-hits-hardest-informal-sector

The World Trade Organization. (2021). *COVID-19 and its effect on Nepal*. Retrieved from https://www.wto.org/english/tratop_e/covid19_e/sawdf_nepal_e.pdf

Tshering, S., & Nima, D. (2021). Bhutan: The role of the constitutional monarch in a public health crisis. In V. Ramraj (Ed.), *COVID-19 in Asia: Law and policy contexts* (pp. 279–282). Oxford University Press. Retrieved November 25, 2021, from https://academic.oup.com/book/33490/chapter/287789665.

Ugyel, I. (2021). *Moving on from the pandemic in Bhutan*. Asia and Pacific Policy Society - Australian National University. Retrieved from https://www.policyforum.net/moving-on-from-the-pandemic-in-bhutan/

UNOCHA. (2021). *Nepal: COVID-19 pandemic situation report no. 49 (As of 1 November 2021)*. Retrieved from https://reliefweb.int/report/nepal/nepal-covid-19-pandemic-situation-report-no-49-1-november-2021

Whitecross, R. (2021). Bhutan in 2020: Controlling the pandemic. *Asian Survey*, *61*(1), 207–210. Retrieved November 25, 2021, from https://online.ucpress.edu/as/article-abstract/61/1/207/116350/Bhutan-in-2020Controlling-the-Pandemic?redirectedFrom=fulltext

World Health Organisation. (2022). *Nepal: WHO coronavirus disease (COVID-19) dashboard with vaccination data*. Retrieved March 7, 2022, from https://covid19.who.int/region/searo/country/np

World Vision. (2021). Multi-sectoral impact of the COVID-19 second wave in Nepal - 2021. Retrieved from https://www.wvi.org/publications/policy-paper/nepal/multi-sectoral-impact-covid-19-second-wave-nepal-2021

Xinhua News Agency. (2021). Bhutan receives 400,000 doses of COVID-19 vaccine from India. Retrieved March 7, 2022, from http://www.xinhuanet.com/english/asiapacific/2021-03/22/c_139827645.htm

5

GLOBAL PANDEMIC'S IMPACT ON THE SECURITY LANDSCAPE

The Transition from the Physical to the Online and the Hybrid Domains

Liu Chunlin and Rohan Gunaratna

5.1 The Shift from the Physical to the Online and the Hybrid Domains

The security environment has seen substantial changes as a result of the global COVID-19 pandemic. Physical security has given way to online and hybrid realms as remote work and online communication have become increasingly mainstream. The convergence of the real and digital worlds exemplifies how we have adapted to new ways of operating. The blending of the real and digital worlds is likely to accelerate as we move into a post-pandemic scenario, bringing both opportunities and challenges.

The globalization of the digital revolution was expedited by the COVID-19 pandemic that struck the world in 2020. The rapid adoption of digital technologies, necessitated by the virus's spread, forced businesses and governments to embrace digital solutions to maintain operational efficiency. Many of these adjustments facilitated the swift implementation of technological advances that would have otherwise taken much longer. The era when personnel were assigned physical office spaces and cabins, and teams assembled in person, has largely given way to a new norm. The introduction of digital workspaces, unprecedented before the pandemic, has marked a new phase of the digital revolution.

Businesses and academic institutions have initiated work-from-home policies in response to heightened digitalization. The growing significance of blockchain technology has prompted the need for comprehensive design and regulatory assessments. Concurrently, the expansion of digital presence has brought attention to concerns regarding workplace surveillance and technostress. Consequently, the adoption of numerous new platforms and technologies has ensued, raising potential security vulnerabilities due to inadequate scrutiny.

DOI: 10.4324/9781003569084-6

Lockdown measures have triggered a notable increase in the utilization of networks and information systems, accompanied by significant shifts in usage habits and behaviours. Individuals are adjusting to a new "normal" where meetings have transitioned entirely online and office tasks are conducted from home, leading to the emergence of novel work patterns. These developments have impacted a wide array of organizations across industry, society, and government. Furthermore, these changes have transpired swiftly, leaving organizations limited time to plan and implement new setups and arrangements. Consequently, they have been compelled to adapt, explore innovative approaches, experiment, and devise solutions previously deemed unattainable.

Amid COVID-19 conditions, various industries and governments exhibit differing degrees of digital technology adoption. Factors such as productivity, economic conditions, market characteristics, and the existing level of technological progress and maturity significantly influence this adoption process. Furthermore, the acceleration of digitalization across industries has been facilitated by the capacity for innovation within digital settings and ecosystems. This has led to the creation of new services that cater to existing markets or even carve out entirely new market segments.

Physical interactions are minimized, and for many organizations, digital connections have become their lifeline. The true meaning of being digital is made evident by COVID-19. It involves having a deep solution chain across processes, people, and technology, not just having cool apps. It represents a major shift in how we conduct business, live, and work. The interplay of scientific and technological progress with digital resources has shown the ability to coordinate efforts to better manage the pandemic's consequences and avoid them.

Looking at the case of Philippines, numerous tech companies were able to allow transition to remote work with ease due to their prior use of various technologies for task completion, even before the pandemic. Moreover, after COVID-19 protocols were relaxed, many businesses chose to continue employing remote workers, citing reasons such as higher productivity and lower costs associated with renting office space. The transition during the lockdown was also manageable for some academic institutions, as they had already begun using the hybrid method and tools like Canvas, Moodle, and Microsoft Teams before the epidemic. In fact, several institutions still conduct the majority of their classes off-site and plan to continue doing so indefinitely.

The associated security threats cannot be disregarded. For example, a corporation mandated that all work be completed in the office despite lockdowns and other regulations, as employees are not permitted to take any sensitive information outside of the workplace. Additionally, some businesses are compelled to utilize GPS to track the whereabouts of their personnel because they cannot allow certain staff to work remotely outside of the Philippines for tax-related reasons. The nation is also becoming increasingly aware that the way these technologies are employed can endanger human-centred values as well as consumer protection, privacy, and security.

Studies have shown that remote work can be more productive than in-office work. For instance, a study by Stanford University found that remote workers were 13% more productive than their in-office counterparts. This increased productivity is attributed to remote workers experiencing fewer distractions and being able to focus on their tasks without interruptions. Hybrid work models allow companies to harness the productivity benefits of remote work while still maintaining the advantages of in-office collaboration and communication.

Several companies have already embraced hybrid work. For example, X platform announced in May 2020 that its employees could work from home permanently if they wanted to (Brian Fung, 2020). Similarly, Shopify, a Canadian e-commerce company, announced that its employees could work from home indefinitely. Other companies, like Microsoft, are adopting a more flexible approach, allowing employees to work from home up to 50% of the time.

Despite these challenges, it is clear that hybrid work is here to stay. The pandemic forced companies to adapt to remote work, and many have found that it to be a viable and beneficial option. By adopting a hybrid approach, companies can offer their employees flexibility while still maintaining the benefits of in-office collaboration and communication.

The transition to remote work has coincided with a rise in the utilization of cloud-based platforms for data processing and collaboration. Although these services have many advantages, they also present new security threats, as sensitive data is now being housed outside an organization's internal network. Digital technology use is growing rapidly, and with it, so are online fraud, scams, invasions, and security breaches. Moreover, the sophistication and focus of these attacks has increased. The administration and control of the internet constitute a crucial component of this increase in digitalization. Despite the fact that the internet is a worldwide resource and no one nation has the power to regulate its protocols and features, local access and availability are still national issues. Nations can act as intermediaries in matters of monitoring, bandwidth restriction, security, intermediary liability, and online transactions.

As more consumers utilize digital technologies, there is an increased risk of cyberattacks and data leaks, jeopardizing the security of sensitive data. The massive rise of electronic and virtual interactions during the pandemic has underscored the importance of securing personal and commercial data. A hybrid security landscape that integrates physical and cybersecurity has also emerged as a result of the epidemic. For instance, businesses and organizations are increasingly employing technology like biometric identification, security cameras, and access control systems to keep an eye on employees and visitors in both real-world and virtual settings.

Security experts now face new hurdles due to the combination of physical and cybersecurity, as they must monitor and address threats in both domains. Cybersecurity has become a primary focus. Since the pandemic, organizations face several security threats that need to be addressed to safeguard their operations and data. By implementing robust security policies and procedures, providing protected access

to company information and networks, minimizing the use of personal devices, and analysing employee behaviour, organizations can reduce the risk of cyber threats and ensure the security of their operations.

In conclusion, the worldwide pandemic has significantly altered the security landscape, prompting a transition to online and hybrid realms. Physical security remains crucial despite the growing reliance on digital technology, which has introduced new security challenges. Security professionals now face both new opportunities and problems due to the convergence of physical and digital security, requiring them to be flexible and adopt new methods and technologies. Overall, the integration and interface of digital platforms during and after COVID-19 introduced new security vulnerabilities for which institutions were unprepared. Due to the rapid rise in cybersecurity events, organizations had to act rapidly to reduce their risks and safeguard their sensitive data.

5.2 Implementation by Security Industry

The convergence of cyber and physical security has become increasingly important in recent years, as threats to both areas have become more sophisticated and interconnected. Cybersecurity focuses on protecting digital assets, such as information stored on computer systems and networks, while physical security focuses on protecting physical assets, such as buildings, people, and equipment.

The impact of this convergence on organizations and security companies can be significant. On one hand, it can increase the effectiveness of security measures by creating a more holistic approach that addresses vulnerabilities in both digital and physical spaces. This can help prevent attacks that exploit the weaknesses in one area to gain access to the other.

On the other hand, the convergence of cyber and physical security can also create new challenges. For example, finding personnel with expertise in both areas can be difficult, potentially resulting in gaps in security measures. Additionally, the convergence of cyber and physical security requires new technologies and processes, which can be expensive and time-consuming to implement.

Overall, the impact of cyber and physical security convergence depends on how well organizations and security companies can adapt to the new challenges and opportunities presented by this trend. Those that successfully integrate cyber and physical security measures can reap significant benefits in terms of improved security and reduced risk.

5.2.1 Connected Operating Environment

Today's threats stem from hybrid attacks targeting both physical and cyber assets. The widespread adoption and integration of Internet of Things (IoT) and Industrial Internet of Things (IIoT) devices have led to an increasingly interconnected mesh of cyber–physical systems (CPS), expanding the attack surface and blurring the once distinct domains of cybersecurity and physical security. Moreover, endeavours to enhance cyber resilience and expedite the adoption of advanced technologies can inadvertently introduce or amplify security risks within this evolving threat landscape.

5.2.2 Integrated Security Strategies

a The overall security protection plan shall prescribe an effective and holistic security protection strategy that includes four levels of integrations:

i Level 1: Integrated electronic systems

Many electronic security systems function as standalone systems, such as CCTV, access control systems, intrusion alarms, and scanners, etc. Integrating these systems enables data analysis, identification of gaps, and enhancement of overall security system performance.

Many business operations depend on electronic security systems to authenticate or verify the employees' identities. For instance, staff cafeteria, wardrobe conveyor, transportation systems, and computer system may need to integrate with the physical access control system for employee authentication. Analysing the data generated from these integrations can provide valuable insights to enhance both operations and security.

ii Level 2: Integrated physical security elements

All elements of physical security must be integrated to function as part of a comprehensive strategy. These elements encompass architecture and engineering, physical barriers and means, procedural controls, deployment and response of security personnel, and various types of electronic security systems. Integration of these measures enhances effectiveness and acts as a force multiplier.

iii Level 3: Integrated security programs

Physical security constitutes just one facet of an overarching protection strategy. Many organizations compartmentalize various security disciplines, leading to redundant resources, inefficient operations and increased overheads. Integration of physical security with other security disciplines such as personnel security, IT security, information security, investigations, executive protection is essential to optimize resources and achieve better results.

iv Level 4: Integration of enterprise risk management

The broadest level of integrated asset protection is at the enterprise level, achieved through the implementation of the enterprise security risk management (ESRM) approach. ESRM aligns security initiatives with the organizational mission, vision, values, and objectives.

5.3 Convergence of Security Solutions

In assets protection, convergence generally means the integration of traditional and IT security functions. A broader definition might consider convergence to be the merging of disciplines, techniques, and tools from various fields for the purpose of protecting critical assets. It is widely accepted that "companies' assets are now increasingly information-based and intangible, and even most physical assets rely heavily on information" (ASIS, 2005). An approach using only physical, or IT security measures is insufficient. Assets protection managers must also employ traditional information security, personnel security, technical security, and public relations and other external communications to protect intangible assets. A true convergence approach would also employ security architecture and design, crime prevention through environmental design, investigations, policies and procedures, and awareness training.

To prepare for the future of cyber and physical security convergence, security companies should take the following steps.

5.3.1 Invest in Training and Education

As cyber and physical security become more intertwined, it is crucial for security companies to cultivate employees with expertise in both areas. Facility management contends with staffing shortage and requires constant training and retraining due to high staff turnover. This can be achieved through training and education programs that teach employees how to identify and address vulnerabilities in both digital and physical environments.

Simultaneously, there is a **pressing need to address this niche and devote energy to train new cybersecurity staff who are ready to deal with emerging complex cyber and physical threats**.

Universities collaborating with the private sector could help address the need for affordable, cutting-edge, large-scale training schemes for cybersecurity experts and practitioners.[1] Similarly, polytechnics should offer cybersecurity courses for talents to be nurtured at younger ages.

5.3.2 Embrace New Technologies

The convergence of cyber and physical security necessitates the adoption of new technologies and tools. Security companies must remain open to adopting these new technologies and exploring how they can be used to enhance security measures.

Furthermore, it should also be ensured that **novel cyber–physical capabilities are tested and secured**. At the same time, innovative developments should be deployed safely.

5.3.3 Develop a Holistic Approach

Cyber and physical security should be regarded as integral components of a broader security ecosystem, rather than isolated areas of concern. Security companies should adopt a holistic approach to security that acknowledges the interdependence between digital and physical systems.

The significance of cyber–physical convergence is widely recognized. On one hand, incident information substantiates that violent non-state actors tend to resort to traditional means. On the other hand, the expansion of digital presence underscores the need for heightened cybersecurity measures due to increased exposure to cyber risks. Nonetheless, given that humans are often the weakest link, **particular emphasis should be placed on the human factor in counter policies**.[2]

Using psychological techniques, it should be made sure that signs of dissatisfaction are identified in a timely manner because people prefer to work from home and spend much less time at the workplace. Since they might be more likely to act maliciously in an unsupervised setting, the screening procedure principles need to be re-examined.[3]

Despite the fact that the pandemic encouraged employees to work from home, and even "stay at home," it is noticeable that numerous companies do not **provide a cyber-safe remote working environment**. It is of great importance to acknowledge that individuals working at home do not enjoy the same level of inherent protection or deterrent measures as they do in a traditional office environment. Once corporate data is accessible from a personal device, cyber risks should be reassessed. At the same time, it is highly advisable that remote working practices are made resilient to cyberattacks.[4]

Good cyber hygiene and practices should be promoted among employees[5] for adaptability and flexibility.

The increased **use of personal cloud storage** should be involved in security policies.[6]

The prevalence of online meetups instead of the previous personal negotiations create novel security-related vulnerabilities.[7]

Secured-remote access solutions (remote monitoring) to observe locations remotely offered significant value during the pandemic times and therefore gained popularity. These solutions will likely remain as primary or secondary options versus physical locations. The evolution of these cloud-based systems should be considered when examining the vulnerabilities of security systems.[8]

Novelties in general and every-day practices (e.g., online shopping experience, QR-code payments) should be noted and the associated risks taken into account.[9]

Risk assessment is to be reconsidered based upon these novel vulnerabilities.

5.3.1 Foster Collaboration

Collaboration between different departments and stakeholders within an organization is crucial for the success of cyber and physical security convergence. Security companies should actively encourage collaboration among IT, physical security, and other relevant departments to identify vulnerabilities and develop effective security strategies.

Companies should take a proactive approach to address the security threats and develop strategies to prevent cyberattacks rather than merely responding to incidents. The **best practices should be consistently gathered to learn from the case studies of other nations**, and successful counter strategies should be applied to address these identified vulnerabilities.[10]

In order to learn from other countries' case studies, best practices should be regularly collected. Successful counterstrategies should then be implemented to address these weaknesses.

Networking among different domains of security is critical. Collaboration between experts on physical infrastructure and professionals in the cybersecurity sector is essential for developing novel approaches and solutions. It is important to **nurture a multi-stakeholder digital security ecosystem** to facilitate the sharing of information.

The crisis situation during the pandemic underscored the importance of national-centric standpoints and led to the closure of borders. Therefore, **it is imperative to reinforce transnational alliances.**

5.3.5   Stay Informed

Finally, security companies should stay informed about the latest trends and developments in both cyber and physical security. This can be achieved through attending conferences, networking with peers, and staying up to date on industry publications and news.

Reportedly, **small businesses** are more vulnerable to cyberattacks. With this in mind, these corporations should also address the associated cyber threats.[11]

Trends of cybersecurity threats should be reviewed; the impacts of, small, medium, and full-scale cyberattacks should be understood.

It is advisable to learn more about international, regional, local security frameworks and measures taken.

Gaps and challenges of adopting integrated physical and cybersecurity, including issues related to manpower, training, retraining, knowledge, research, and development, and government funding should be identified. In parallel, efforts should be made to increase public awareness through education and training on these topics.

5.4   Implementation by Owners/Developers/City Mayors

5.4.1   Existing Physical Security Countermeasures to Be Integrated into Digital Security Systems

Physical security provision is still necessary, but the demand for digital security provisions in development and daily city operations is growing. Major security challenges are likely to arise from the digital world rather than the physical world.

With the implementation of digital solutions such as CCTV and visitor management system, vulnerabilities to cyberattacks become apparent.

The novel and complex security threat landscape requires a holistic approach. An integrated security system ensures a multilevel, enhanced protection against malicious attacks. These layered concepts are tailor-designed according to the novel threat indicators.

5.4.2 Owner/Developer/Mayor to Be Decision Makers for Both Physical World and Digital World

Owners, developers, and city mayors play a crucial role in better understanding and addressing this novel hybrid threat landscape. These stakeholders must adapt to newly emerging threat indicators and adjust their capabilities accordingly. This requires a reconsidered and proactive security approach, along with the planning and implementation of a holistic security system.

5.4.3 Addressing Security Challenges from Both the Digital and the Physical Worlds

Exploring and implementing innovative technologies and solutions are the best option for owners, developers, and mayors to address security threats of both digital and physical nature. Holistic consideration, planning, and implementation are necessary for both physical and cyber protection. By taking the following steps, building owners can help ensure that their buildings are prepared to address both cyber and physical security threats, now and in the future:

5.4.3.1 Conduct a Risk Assessment

Building owners should conduct a comprehensive risk assessment to identify vulnerabilities in both digital and physical systems. This assessment should cover all areas of the building, including the IT infrastructure, building management systems, and physical security measures.

Security consultation with owners and city mayors should begin with detecting novel vulnerabilities in the security system. New practices implemented in the aftermath of the pandemic should be taken into account. Following a thorough examination of these novel vulnerabilities, risk assessments should be reconsidered accordingly.

5.4.3.2 Develop a Comprehensive Security Plan

Based on the results of the risk assessment, building owners should develop a comprehensive security plan that addresses both cyber and physical security concerns. This plan should include measures to prevent, detect, and respond to security incidents.

5.4.3.3   Use Secure Technologies

Building owners should utilize secure technologies designed to address both cyber and physical security concerns. This includes technologies such as access control systems, video surveillance systems, and intrusion detection systems that are designed to integrate with other security systems.

5.4.3.4   Train Building Staff

Training and increasing the security awareness of owners and their staff should be given a particular emphasis.

Building owners should provide training to building staff on how to identify and respond to security threats. This includes training on the effective use of security systems, as well as training on how to identify and report suspicious activity.

5.4.3.5   Work with Security Experts

Building owners should collaborate with security experts who can provide guidance on addressing both cyber and physical security concerns. These experts can help building owners develop and implement effective security measures, as well as offer ongoing support and guidance as security threats evolve over time.

Security consultation should shed light on the potential motives behind physical or cyberattacks, such as financial harm or "hacktivism." This understanding can encourage owners and city mayors to take more proactive and preventative countermeasures.

The holistic nature of physical and cybersecurity should be emphasized for clients, making it a priority to raise their awareness of the significance of this integrated approach.

Clients may be reluctant to allocate a budget for creating and maintaining a safe and secure environment. In practice, they wait until the first harmful incident to devote focused attention to their security. To make them more inclined to take preventive actions, an incident database on malicious acts should be established and consistently maintained. Real-life examples can then be cited to help clients better understand the proximity of the threat.

Once the threat landscape has been meticulously examined, it may be advisable to determine levels of security and accordingly create packages of services (e.g., basic, advanced, superior). Smaller businesses with limited budgets may be more prone to devote at least a minimum attention to ensuring their physical and cybersecurity.

For developers, it is crucial to understand the threat landscape. To achieve this, they need to collaborate closely with clients. In additional, developers must maintain active professional interaction with other experts in the field to ensure that they devise innovative solutions.

5.5 Security and Happiness by Design Approach

"Security and happiness by design" is identified as a paradigm that seeks to integrate elements of happiness with the complexity of physical protection and safety goals throughout the entire process for a facility, from the planning through construction and operation.

Historically, security measures have been established to enhance the physical security of citizens who use these facilities or buildings. However, in reality, the elevated level of security can lead to a less reassured feeling in people living in a space controlled by a multisensory system. Based on two decades of professional experience with clients, K&C Protective Technologies Pte. Ltd. argues that this anxiety should be considered when designing the security of a building.

Therefore, it is advisable that people's happiness becomes a significant factor in the planning process. Incorporating this happiness element would not only increase the sustainability index of a city through high social equity but also, in the long run, meet the social requirements and result in an increased commercial demand.

There have been continuous efforts in security design research. The security system design is the process that allows clients to control the access that people (insiders and outsiders) have to the organization's assets. This coordinated and prioritized approach ensures asset protection by design. The designers need to work with the clients, architects, and engineers to incorporate security elements into the overall corporate facility/campus design. Client outcomes include layers of business security based on the value of the assets, flexibility, efficiencies, and cost savings (Kelling & Coles, 1997), (Liu & Gunaratna, 2021a).

Artificial intelligence and machine learning (AIML) applications should include security systems. Video surveillance, by processing images of people, has proved effective and increasingly used in both public and private domains to prevent and recode crimes (Dambalkar et al., 2020). However, video surveillance recordings may also interfere with the legally protected privacy of individuals, because video surveillance records may involve processing of personal data (Cavallaro, 2007). It is not only about observation and recording of images, but also about their transmission in networks, analysis, storage and archiving of storage devices, as well as destruction of the recordings or the entire storage device. Proposed analysis of statistical data concerning urban video surveillance as a tool to improve the security of public spaces in the city of Katowice was reported in (Socha & Kogut, 2020). The technical and organizational solutions applied, as in the case of the Katowice smart surveillance and analysis system, made it possible to assess the impact of the operation of the system on offenses and the number of legal proceedings.

Psychology is the study of mind and behaviour. The modern security system is a cyber–physical system (CPS). It is the integration of computation, networking, and physical processes. Putting humans in this loop defines a new discipline of CPS called cyber–physical human systems (CPHSs) or human-in-the-loop (Sowe et al.,

2016). Human factors and engineering psychologists study how people interact with machines and technology (Carayon, 2006). They use psychological science to guide the design of products, systems, and devices we use every day. They often focus on performance and safety. The work of human factors affecting adoption of new technologies is most relevant to our work (Taherdoost, 2019). Psychological acceptance is the active embracing of subjective experience, particularly distressing experiences. These tools include mindfulness, cognitive distancing or diffusion, metacognition, experiential or psychological acceptance, psychological flexibility, and meditation (Barnes-Holmes et al., 2001).

Different from the existing approaches, we address the problem by incorporating happiness elements in the design of security systems. The development of security systems and psychology are typically treated as separate research areas, yet they are inherently interconnected. Much can be achieved by combining security and happiness together.

Besides assessment criteria for artificial intelligence, considering happiness elements in the optimized security risk assessment methodology for the building under the blast effect analysis brings novel perspectives into the systematic framework of threat assessment, vulnerability assessment, and consequence (impact) assessment.

Incorporating the happiness elements into a construction process may enhance resistance to blast incidents. For example, building double walls and adding aesthetics such as pictures, green walls, or architectural designs can help people accept these solutions. Meanwhile, reinforced structures with these extraordinary walls substantially increase the blast resistance of the building. Another example is replacing anti-crash bollards systems with planter boxes, chairs/benches or trees, which not only prevent unauthorized vehicle access but also bring joy to visitors and considerably harden malicious access to the building. Green walls, for instance, provide the same security-related advantages as steel plates with reinforced concrete walls, while also igniting pleasant feelings in people passing by.

5.6 The Future

Humans are a social species. Human-to-human interaction was impeded with the pandemic. With the restoration of communication becoming a global imperative both for work and life, there was a global sea change. The pandemic witnessed lounges turning into offices, and bedrooms being used as conference rooms. To survive and sustain businesses during the pandemic required adaption and evolution. The remote model has become the dominant model to restore communication. The lack of effective communication disrupted cooperation, collaboration, and partnership, driving businesses to fail. The challenges of communication were overcome by technology.

A May 2022 study of 125 CEOs and decision makers reported, "Slack is the most popular platform for workplace communication – used by 52% of respondents." This was followed by Zoom (47%), and Google Hangouts/Meet (26%)."[12]

From the remote model, the hybrid model evolved. Hybrid working became the norm during the pandemic, a trend likely to persist. The flexible work environment with remote working was productive, reduced cost, and even improved morale.[13] The model of working in which employees split their time between working remotely and working in the office is the hybrid model.

All surveys found that employees would prefer a hybrid model of working postpandemic. "LinkedIn reports that 87% of employees will want to remain remote most of the time."[14] The Oxford Group's practical guide to managing hybrid teams sought to answer eight key questions that many grapple with to this date.

1 How do you build/maintain trust in your team?
2 How do you ensure you're inclusive?
3 How do you bring somebody new on board?
4 How do you project a vision?
5 How do people learn on the job?
6 How do you manage performance remotely?
7 How do you navigate change?
8 How do you create the right company atmosphere?

"Although teams have been working together remotely, across sites and geographies for a long time, the novelty here is the magnitude of change."[15] After evolving from the remote to the hybrid model, business is now grappling with a realistic model for the future. In developing that realistic model, one of the new challenges the world is experiencing is to create both productive staff with integrity as well as safe and secure technology.

5.7 Conclusion

During and after the COVID-19 pandemic, the boundaries and borders have changed and reshaped our lives. Hybrid schedules have changed and will continue to impact both work and living. New homes will have dedicated workplaces. Work–life balance will need to be maintained to preserve both work integrity and family commitment. The future of work and life will be markedly different from the past and the present. This digital acceleration has not been accompanied by a corresponding security and leadership transformation.

Hybrid work and life in a post-pandemic landscape brings both challenges and opportunities. Billions of people changed their behaviour in countless ways after the pandemic and are engaging in flexible work-life arrangements.[16] Reverting to large offices is unlikely, as employees desire greater autonomy. Sustaining employee morale and productivity is crucial. However, tracking time spent on work through technologies like internet surveillance, cyber monitoring, and keystroke monitoring software may lead to mistrust and paranoia.[17] Instead, monitoring performance by output rather than digital FaceTime may be more effective. When navigating the hybrid world, employees will have to understand the importance of building relationships to ensure work commitment when not present in office.

Although hybrid living minimizes commuting time and reduces the need for large offices, the downside is less human interaction, which is vital for building team spirit and strengthening teamwork. Physical face-to-face interaction is essential for building emotional and personal bonds. Therefore, maintaining collegiality and friendship is as important as ever. The employee approach should prioritize cooperation, collaboration, and partnership through personalization. This entails engaging to instil loyalty, collective decision making, and a far-reaching leadership. What is needed are inspiring words and listening to plan and prepare, rather than measures to compel and coerce a staff to deliver. Leaders at all levels needs to be mindful and strive to be the best trained in patience and ingenuity for engaging staff remotely.

To facilitate hybrid work, government and private sector leadership must address security threats, risks, and challenges. Due to the global surge in remote workers, there has been a "significant scaling up of cyber threats across the board with credential theft and social attacks such as phishing and business email compromises the cause of over 67 per cent of all breaches."[18]

In addition, "Web application breaches doubled, accounting for 43 per cent of all breaches." With the public relying on the online domain for work and life, governments must secure security systems to protect both work and personal data. As staff work from outside their workplaces and access sensitive data, the data will need to be protected. Unless standard security arrangements are in place, it will be like visiting a cyber cafe to use a computer. Not only will both government and the private sector invest more in guiding their staff on cyber hygiene, but governments will need to strengthen their cybersecurity agencies to enhance surveillance and cyber investigative authorities to investigate any breaches.

Change is inevitable. Despite the vast progress of humankind in science and technology in the past century, nature remains the greatest force on earth. To mitigate threats and risks, respect for planet Earth, articulated in all the great faiths, should be the foundation of human living. The sea change after the COVID-19 pandemic demonstrates that the future is in hybrid working and living. To support the paradigm shift in security thinking, planning, and execution, both government and industry leaders should rise to the challenge. To reinforce a smooth transition, technological shift, and mind-set change, the world will witness, in the coming months and years, new approaches to secure the physical, online, and hybrid domains. The seamless function and integration of health and well-being, security and happiness by design will be the defining feature of the new and emerging security architecture.

Notes

1 Organisation for Economic Co-operation and Development (OECD). (n.d.). *Seven lessons learned about digital security during the COVID-19 crisis*. Retrieved December 6, 2024, from https://www.oecd.org/coronavirus/policy-responses/seven-lessons-learned-about-digital-security-during-the-covid-19-crisis-e55a6b9a/

2 KPMG. (2021). *The importance of cyber security in the post-COVID-19 world*. Retrieved December 6, 2024, from https://kpmg.com/mt/en/home/insights/2021/07/the-importance-of-cyber-security-in-the-post-covid19-world.html

3 Security Industry Association. (2023). *Security after COVID-19: A guide to the post-pandemic security industry*. Retrieved December 6, 2024, from https://www.securityindustry.org/wp-content/uploads/2023/02/SIA-Security-After-Covid.pdf

4 Deloitte. (n.d.). *The impact of COVID-19 on cybersecurity*. Retrieved December 6, 2024, fromhttps://www2.deloitte.com/ch/en/pages/risk/articles/impact-covid-cybersecurity.html

5 Gartner. (n.d.). *7 security areas to focus on during COVID-19*. Retrieved December 6, 2024, from https://www.gartner.com/smarterwithgartner/7-security-areas-to-focus-on-during-covid-19

6 Trend Micro. (2021). *Looking ahead: The post-pandemic security landscape*. Retrieved December 6, 2024, from https://www.trendmicro.com/en_us/research/21/f/looking-ahead–the-post-pandemic-security-landscape.html

7 TechTarget. (n.d.). *Cybersecurity lessons learned from COVID-19 pandemic*. Retrieved December 6, 2024, from https://www.techtarget.com/searchsecurity/feature/Cybersecurity-lessons-learned-from-COVID-19-pandemic

8 Berling, T. V. (2021). International organizations and COVID-19: *Managing the crisis or the new normal? European View, 20*(1), 50–58 https://journals.sagepub.com/doi/full/10.1177/17816858211059250

9 Everbridge. (n.d.). *The new normal: Managing physical and digital security threats in a COVID-19 world*. Retrieved December 6, 2024, from https://www.everbridge.com/blog/the-new-normal-managing-physical-and-digital-security-threats-in-a-covid-19-world/

10 Pluralsight. (n.d.). *7 security threats introduced by COVID-19 and the WFH rush*. Retrieved December 6, 2024, from https://www.pluralsight.com/blog/security-professional/-7-security-threats-introduced-by-covid-19-and-the-wfh-rush

11 Stockholm International Water Institute (SIWI). (n.d.). *Don't forget the security aspect of the COVID-19 crisis*. Retrieved December 6, 2024, from https://siwi.org/latest/dont-forget-the-security-aspect-of-the-covid-19-crisis/

12 Expert Market. (n.d.). *11 key workplace communication statistics*. Retrieved December 6, 2024, from https://www.expertmarket.com/phone-systems/workplace-communication-statistics#link-11-key-workplace-communication-statistics

13 Startups Magazine. (n.d.). *Here's how hybrid work has evolved since the pandemic*. Retrieved December 6, 2024, from https://startupsmagazine.co.uk/article-heres-how-hybrid-work-has-evolved-start-pandemic

14 Oxford Group. (n.d.). *The rise of hybrid working: Why it's the future of work*. Retrieved December 6, 2024, from https://www.oxford-group.com/insights/rise-hybrid-working-why-its-future-work

15 Oxford Group. (n.d.). *A practical guide to managing hybrid teams*. Retrieved December 6, 2024, from https://www.oxford-group.com/sites/default/files/PDF/A%20practical%20guide%20to%20managing%20hybrid%20teams%20-%20Pages.pdf

16 McKinsey & Company. (n.d.). *Empty spaces and hybrid places: Chapter 1*. Retrieved December 6, 2024, from https://www.mckinsey.com/mgi/our-research/empty-spaces-and-hybrid-places-chapter-1

17 Singapore Management University. (n.d.). *The future of work: Why the hybrid model is here to stay*. Retrieved December 6, 2024, from https://business.smu.edu.sg/mba/lkcsb-community/future-work-hybrid-model-here-stay

18 Financial Times. (n.d.). *The security challenges of hybrid working*. Retrieved December 6, 2024, from https://www.ft.com/partnercontent/verizon/the-security-challenges-of-hybrid-working.html

Bibliography

ASIS International. (2005). "Companies' assets are now increasingly information-based and intangible, and even most physical assets rely heavily on information".

Barnes-Holmes, Y., Steven, C. H., Dermot, B.-H., & Roche, B. (2001). *Relational frame theory: A post-Skinnerian account of human language and cognition*. Plenum Press.

Brian Fung. (2020). "Twitter will let some employees work from home forever," CNN Business, May 2020 Bottom of Form.

Carayon, P. (2006). Human factors of complex sociotechnical systems. *Applied Ergonomics, 37*(4), 525–535.

Cavallaro, A. (2007). Privacy in video surveillance. *IEEE Signal Processing Magazine, 24*(2), 168–166.

Dambalkar, P., Gupta, A., Pande, A., & Ladekar, A. (2020). Smart surveillance system – Literature survey. *International Research Journal of Engineering and Technology (IRJET), 7*(5), 15–24.

Kelling, G. L., & Coles, C. M. (1997). *Fixing broken windows: Restoring order and reducing crime in our communities*. Simon and Schuster.

K. Sowe, S., Koji, Z., Simmon, E., de Vaulx, F., & Bojanova, I. (2016). Cyber-physical human systems: Putting people in the loop. *IT Professional, 18*(1), 10–13.

Liu, C.-L., & Gunaratna, R. (2021a). Lebanon's single most destructive explosion – Terrorists plan to copy and provision against such accidents. *Journal of Applied Security Research, 3*, 1–22.

Liu, C.-L., & Gunaratna, R. (2021b). The terrorist threat forecast in 2021. *Revista UNISCI/UNISCI Journal, 55*, 215–220.

Socha, R., & Kogut, B. (2020). Urban video surveillance as a tool to improve security in public spaces. *Sustainability, 12*(15), 6210.

Taherdoost, H. (2019). A review of technology acceptance and adoption models and theories. *Procedia Manufacturing, 22*, 960–967.

6

CYBERSECURITY AND CYBERCRIME IN THE MENA

Kyounggun Kim

6.1   Introduction

The Middle East and North Africa (MENA) region is a very important region that connects three continents: Africa, Asia, and Europe. The MENA region is moving forwards as a digital society more than at any other time in history. The world has inevitably demanded a change to a digital society according to the changes of the times. Although the change to a digital society has many advantages, new threats to countries, companies, and individuals such as cybercrime and cyberattacks arise. In this paper, we propose focusing on cooperation, capability, and assessment (CCA) for cybersecurity and cybercrime in the MENA region. We hope that these important factors will help maintain the ongoing cybersecurity and international peace of the MENA.

6.2   Connecting the World

After the end of World War II, the US Department of Defense considered how to manage information continuously for the purpose of keeping information safe in the event of a nuclear war. In 1969, the US Department of Defense's Advanced Research Project Administration (ARPA) initiated a study on exchanging information between distant systems for the safe preservation of information. As a result, ARPANET, the first network, was created by connecting the University of California, Los Angeles, Stanford Research Institute (SRI), the University of California, Santa Barbara, and the University of Utah. South Korea is the second country in the world to successfully connect to the network. In May 1982, Seoul National University and the Electronics and Telecommunications Research Institute established a network connection network through their own development.

DOI: 10.4324/9781003569084-7

ARPANET was originally the first network created for military purposes, but as a need arose from the private sector, the Ministry of Defense created a separate MILNET, and the National Science Foundation (NSF) built and operated a new communications network in 1986. Since then, in 1987, the new communication network replaced ARPANET as the backbone network of the Internet. At this time, the network was also used for a small number of military or research purposes and was not open to the public.

In 1989, Tim Burners-Lee of CERN, The European Organization for Nuclear Research, studied a way to easily share information scattered across multiple organizations. Through this, the World Wide Web (WWW) was born. The first Internet web site was http://info.cern.ch/hypertext/WWW/TheProject.html, which was released to the public in January 1991. From this point on, the world's Internet connection began.

In the MENA region, Saudi Arabia first started Internet connectivity in 1993 at the College of Computer Sciences and Engineering of King Fahd University of Petroleum and Minerals (KFUPM). Later, in 1995, the King Abdulaziz City for Science and Technology (KACST) provided an Internet channel of 64 Kbps to King Faisal Specialist Hospital and Research Center (KSHRC) and KFUPM. In 1998, KACST provided Internet service with Saudi Telecommunications Company (STC).

In Saudi Arabia, the number of Internet users grew from 100,000 in 1999 to 1 million in 2001 and 31.8 million in 2020, with 91.5% of the total population using the Internet. Not only Saudi Arabia, but also other countries such as the UAE have seen a rapid increase in Internet usage since 2000.

Among the MENA region countries, Qatar (104.3%), UAE (103.3%), Kuwait (98.3%), Bahrain (97.7%), Iran (91.8%), and Saudi Arabia (90.1%) are the top countries with the highest Internet usage as of 2021. On the other hand, the lowest countries are Yemen (25.9%), Syria (46.5%)y and Egypt (52.5%).

In this way, in the MENA region, only 30 years after the Internet was created, many citizens are accessing information through the Internet in cyberspace and engaging in various activities.

6.3   Cyberattacks and Cybercrime in the MENA Region

As Internet users increase and change to a digital society, crimes that disturb the existing social order are naturally occurring on the Internet and digital society. According to Salem Fadi, the top five concerns of Internet users in the region are 1) cyberterrorism, 2) cybercrimes, 3) cyberbullying, 4) "fake news" online, and 5) commercial exploitation of Internet users. Over 40% of users cited these threats as "very" concerning." Cyberterrorism is one of the biggest concerns in the region: 81% of Internet users in the region are concerned about cyberterrorism; 75% of Internet users in the region express online cybercrimes as their second major concern. About 75% of users reported experiencing at least one cyberthreat in the past two years (2015–2017).

Saudi Arabia is undergoing a transformation into a digital nation as part of its national strategy: Saudi Vision 2030. With the catchphrase "Digital Saudi," national digital transformation is in progress. According to the Global Competitiveness Report 2019 for the internet use, UAE ranks 25th, Saudi Arabia 36th, Qatar 29th, Bahrain 45th, Kuwait 46th, Oman 53rd, Jordan 70th, Morocco 75th, Tunisia 87th, Lebanon 88th, Algeria 89th, Egypt 93rd, and Yemen 140th. On the other hand, many countries in Europe and Asia show a fairly high level, with Singapore at first, 2nd place is the United States, 3rd place Hong Kong, 4th place Netherlands, 5th place Switzerland, 6th place Japan, 7th place Germany, 8th place Sweden, 9th place United Kingdom, and 10th place Denmark.

With the Fourth Industrial Revolution discussed at the World Economic Forum, digital transformation is going more powerfully around the world. The UN 2030 Agenda of Sustainable Development, for example, states that digital technologies are essential to achieving Sustainable Development Goals (SDG). However, the UN also highlights some of the threats and risks arising from digital transformation.

There are many actors who disturb the security of the digital society. To keep cyberspace safe, there needs to be awareness about cyberattackers. Cyberattackers have a variety of actors, from curious script kids to cyberterrorists, cybercriminals, and state-sponsored hackers. Cyberthreat actors are threatening cyberspace in a wide range from financial gains to the destruction of national digital infrastructure networks.

In Sameh Aboul-Enein's paper, the importance of cyberwarfare and doctrines is recognized from the perspective of global military power, and many countries are reinforcing these capabilities. Non-state actors are also becoming very familiar with exploiting cyber vulnerabilities. Advances in cyberwarfare and offensive cyber technologies are further fueling this competitive environment. The relevance of existing international humanitarian laws on the use of force in cyberspace, and the obligations of states and international institutions to do so, are becoming ever greater. Sameh Aboul-Enein describes four key challenges for cybersecurity in the Middle East: (i) economics, (ii) education and the Internet gender gap, (iii) cybercrime, and (iv) cyberterrorism and the threat to nuclear security. He mentions the different economic levels of countries in the Middle East, and thus the limitations of resources to counter cybercrime and cyberterrorism. He also emphasizes the importance of Internet gender gap and education. He emphasizes the need for ICT education and the enactment of cyber-related laws to better respond to cyberterrorism and cybercrime. He noted that Arab stakeholders should strengthen the cyber security culture for individual, national, and international security.

The losses to the national economy and corporations due to cybercrime are increasing very significantly. In December 2020, FireEye was attacked, causing corporate stock prices to plummet, and critical information related to national security was leaked. The countries in the MENA region are at the top of the international financial crime statistics. These statistics indicate that about 63% of business enterprises in the region are exposed to economic cybercrime. A more serious problem is that, according to a 2016 survey by PricewaterhouseCoopers (PwC), about 21% of respondents did not even know that their organization was harmed by cybercrime. Another 42% of respondents said that these cyberattacks have caused high- or medium-level damage to their business reputation. According to a survey by PWC, financial losses incurred by cyberattacks and cybercrime in the MENA region amounted to US$5 million–$100 million.

According to a report published by the UN Broadband Commission, 75% of women experienced cyber violence online. Online abuses for women include hate speech, hacking, identity theft, and online stalking, and human trafficking.

Terrorist organizations and non-state actors are using cyber technology as propaganda tools for their goals. Because cyberspace is highly anonymous, it is difficult to trace the origin of the attacker. Cyberterrorist organizations heavily use cyber tools to recruit young people by exploiting anti-establishment sentiments. State-sponsored attacks are consistent with political, social, and military gains. Gauss, a complex cyber-espionage toolkit, conducted cyberattacks against financial institutions in Lebanon, and Flame was used to cyber-espionage against private institutions and universities in Syria, Lebanon, and Saudi Arabia (The National, 2012). These tools could turn on the camera on the victim's device and intercept conversations or keyboard input.

Thus, many serious damages have occurred to individuals, companies, and countries from various and organized cyberattacks such as cybercriminals and cyberterrorists. Sometimes simple but high-impact cyberthreats also arise. Although many efforts are being made to cope with such cybercrimes and cyberthreats such as cyberterrorists, there is still a lack of systematic strategies and policies to prevent and respond to them. Therefore, in the MENA region, cyber diagnosis at the national level is necessary to protect the cybersecurity and important information of citizens, companies, and countries from various cyberthreat actors. In addition, cooperation from MENA region and systematic cybersecurity talent training are needed.

6.4   Cyberterrorists

Cyberterrorism mainly refers to terrorism occurring in cyberspace. The purpose of terrorism is to create fear and terror in the public for a specific purpose. The purpose of cyberterrorists is to create some form of fear and horror to the public through computer technology. The most representative example of cyberterrorism is the "Fire Sale Attack." In the 2007 film *Die Hard 4*, cyberterrorists destroyed the national infrastructure in three stages. The first step is to paralyze all traffic systems. It neutralizes all traffic systems such as road signals, railway lines, subway systems, and aviation systems. And the second step destroys the financial system: delete Wall Street, banking, and financial information. And the third is to destroy public industrial systems such as electricity, water, gas, communications, and satellite systems.

There has been an incident, which seems to come out of the movie, in which a cyberterrorist was arrested in the real world. In 2015, a radical Sunni armed group, Iraq-Levantian Islamic State (ISIL), hacked the personal information of U.S. soldiers and federal government officials in the US Justice Department. A European Kosovo citizen named Ardit Ferizi was confirmed and arrested. Through this incident, we can see that dangerous terrorist organizations in the real world hire or recruit hackers in the form of contracts and require them to bring information to their advantage.

According to a US government agency site (https://www.state.gov/foreign-terrorist-organizations/), as of May 2021, terrorist organizations worldwide are known to the public. A total of 72 are listed, ranging from Boko Haram to unfamiliar groups. One of the most radical terrorist groups, the Iraqi-Syrian Islamic State (ISIS), hired Indian hackers in 2006 to hack government websites and then required $10,000 per hack as a condition for the government to recover information. Hamas, a Palestinian armed organization, created its own cyberterrorist group, Izad-Dean al-Kasam's Cyber Warriors, and launched a distributed denial of service (DDoS) attack against Bank of America (BOA), BB&T, JP Morgan Chase, and the New York Stock Exchange. In 2017, the United Cyber Khalifa (UCC), an IS-linked hacking organization, released a list of 8786 US and British people, including President Donald Trump, instructing lonely wolf terrorists around the world to kill anyone on the list as soon as they see it. Although the biggest target for cyber terrorists is government agencies, the terrorists' greatest purpose is to instill fear in the public, such as in the London subway terrorism and the terrorist attacks in Paris, France, so the activities of cyber terrorists who support the purpose are ultimately against civilians The damage is to the people.

6.5 Tools Used By Cybercriminals and Cyberterrorists

6.5.1 Ransomware and Cryptocurrency

Ransomware (ransom software) is a type of malware designed to encrypt valuable data until a requested ransom amount from the attacker is satisfied. Numerous incidents include Fortune 500 companies, banks, cloud providers, chip manufacturers, cruise operators, threat monitoring services, governments, medical centers and hospitals, schools, universities, and even police departments. The total loss to organizations due to ransomware will be around $20 billion in 2021, and it is expected that a new organization will be hit by an attack every 11 seconds. Worse than that, In 2020, the first loss of human life because of ransomware attacks was reported to take place in Germany. Cybercriminals have perfected ransomware attack components (e.g., stronger encryption techniques, pseudo-anonymous payment methods, worm-like capabilities, etc.), and even started to provide ransomware as a service (RaaS).

Attack phases of ransomware are as follows: (i) infection: in this phase, ransomware is delivered to a victim's system; (ii) communication with command and control (C&C) servers: ransomware connects to the C&C server to exchange crucial information (i.e., encryption keys, target system information) with the attacker; (iii) destruction: ransomware performs the actual malicious actions such as encrypting files; and (iv) extortion: ransomware informs the victim about the attack by displaying a ransom note.

6.5.2   Ransomware as a Service (RaaS) in 2015

RaaS aimed to provide user-friendly and easy-to-modify ransomware kits that could be purchased by anyone on underground markets. In 2017, WannaCry became the main protagonist of the worst cybercrime of that year. It affected more than 250,000 systems in 150 countries. It used AES to encrypt each file with a different key, then individual keys were encrypted using a 2048-bit RSA, a type of asymmetric cryptographic algorithm.

Ransomware can employ symmetric, asymmetric, or hybrid encryption techniques. In symmetric-key encryption only one key is used to encrypt and decrypt files. Advanced encryption standard (AES) is the most popular algorithm. In asymmetric-key encryption, ransomware utilizes a pair of keys, namely public and private keys, to encrypt and decrypt files. Ransomware first uses symmetric key encryption to encrypt victim's files quickly. After that, it encrypts the used symmetric key with the attacker's public key.

6.6   Recommendations for Security in the MENA Region

People in the MENA region are now getting used to the Internet and digital society, and the government is growing one step further with the change to a digital society. In addition to this, cyber threats are also increasing, so to keep the MENA region safe and peaceful from various cyber threats, we propose focusing on the cooperation, capability, and assessment (CCA) approach. Additionally, this method can be performed in top-down, bottom-up, short-term, and long-term (TBSL) ways (Figure 6.1).

6.6.1   Cooperation-Driven (Top-Down Approach)

Cyberthreat actors have no national boundaries. Cyberattacks do not occur only in one country, but often occur simultaneously in multiple countries. Cooperation between countries is essential to proactively respond to various cyberthreats such as cybercriminals and cyberterrorists and to show rapid recovery resilience.

The United States and Europe established the North Atlantic Treaty Organization (NATO) in 1949 and are engaged in joint military response activities. In 2007, in Tallinn, capital of Estonia, as the national infrastructure collapsed due to a cyberattack, it became clear that cyberattacks were a serious threat to the country. Later, in 2008, the NATO Cooperative Cyber Defense Center of Excellence (CCDCOE) was created as a joint cybersecurity cooperative organization against cyberattacks. NATO CCDCOE conducts exchanges and joint research with experts through Cyber Conflict (CyCon) in Tallinn, Estonia every year.

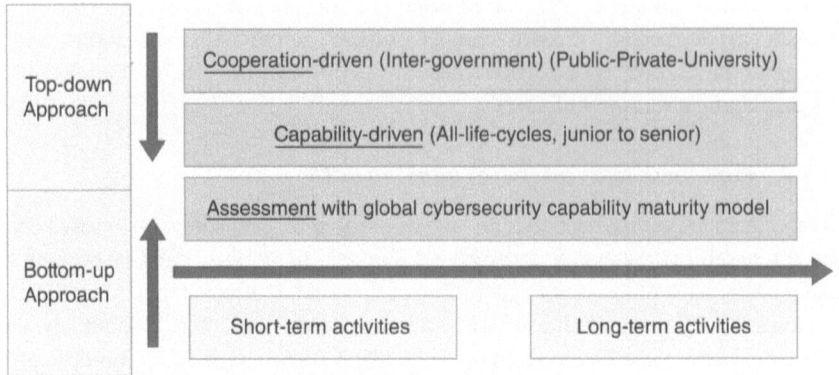

FIGURE 6.1   Proposed approach of Cooperation, Capability, and Assessment (ACC) approach performed in top-down, bottom-up, short-term, and long-term (**TBSL**)

Source: Author's own work.

The European Union issued a joint statement in 2017 titled "Resilience, Defense and Defense: Building strong cybersecurity for the EU." Through a joint statement, EU countries are promoting activities such as strengthening the European Union's level of resilience against cyberattacks, strengthening detection capabilities against cyberattacks, and strengthening international cooperation on cybersecurity (Al-Tawil, 2001). For these activities, the European Union has secured its position as the European Union Agency for Cybersecurity (ENISA), a specialized cybersecurity agency, and has forced ENISA to carry out various cybersecurity activities in the European Union.

6.6.2 Assessment with Global Cybersecurity Capability Maturity Model (Bottom-Up Approach)

The cybersecurity of the MENA region requires a meticulous assessment of the current situation above all else. It is difficult to effectively allocate time and financial support without specific details on which cyberthreat actors and which assets should be protected. Therefore, it is necessary to proceed with accurate assessment with a bottom-up strategy. We must find what is missing and fill the gap. This requires a full national and regional cybersecurity assessment. Areas such as policy, people, process, and technology should be assessed. It should be systematically assessed through joint cybersecurity research and cooperation among the MENA countries mentioned above. There are two approaches for national and regional cybersecurity assessment.

The first is to assess with a well-known model. The second method is to develop a customized cybersecurity capability maturity model based on the characteristics of the MENA region, distribute it to MENA countries, receive opinions, and develop continuously (NDTAR, 2019). Through this, it is possible to assess the current cybersecurity status of MENA countries, to suggest ways to go further, and to continuously monitor and manage.

Among the known models, there is the Cybersecurity Capability Maturity Model for Nations made by the United Nations. There are five areas of maturity models: D1. cybersecurity policy and strategy; D2. cyber culture and society; D3. cybersecurity education, training, and skills; D4. legal and regulatory framework; and D5. standards organizations and technology. Based on this, each country should establish a cybersecurity national strategy, and the national strategy should be aligned with the common values of MENA countries.

There is also an evaluation and analysis method according to the Global Cybersecurity Index developed by ITU-T (Barclay, 2014). The UK also created the Global Cyber Security Capacity Center to develop, evaluate, and manage indicators.

Organization need to measure, evaluate, and continuously manage this way. In addition, it is necessary to make efforts to grow one step further through the evaluation among MENA countries, and through workshops and exchanges of various experts in areas that are mutually insufficient. As the GCSCC evaluation model was also developed by a group of 50 experts, it is necessary to gather experts from MENA countries to create a national cybersecurity maturity evaluation model that fits the characteristics of MENA countries. In the US, former President Joe Biden invested $9 billion to strengthen US cybersecurity capabilities, strengthening the work of the US Cybersecurity and Information Security Administration (CISA) and expanding security upgrades across the federation.

Since the MENA region has a large difference in economic levels between countries, leading countries in the MENA are led by sharing digital transformation, cybersecurity policy, strategy, evaluation, and diagnosis and helping MENA countries grow and develop together. For joint cybersecurity and peace in MENA countries, more advanced MENA countries first preemptively develop a cybersecurity evaluation model and a gap analysis model, and spread them to the remaining MENA countries, and a joint peace and cybersecurity system should be built. Through this, it is possible to reduce the risk of cyberterrorism and cybercrime, and to prevent and respond more rapidly.

6.6.3 Assessment with Global Cybersecurity Capability Maturity Model (Bottom-Up Approach)

In cybersecurity, the balance of hard power and soft power is essential. Human capital skills are crucial in soft power. Cybersecurity problems cannot be resolved in a short period of time and will continue to arise in the future. Therefore, it is necessary to train cybersecurity experts to strengthen cybersecurity capabilities. It is not a short-term approach to nurturing talent, but a mid- to long-term and continuous approach. From children to undergraduates, masters, doctors, and specialized companies, education and training must be conducted to cultivate personnel and to continuously strengthen competence. And such training should be developed and carried out in accordance with the cybersecurity strategy of not only individual MENA countries but also the MENA region.

To cultivate cyber experts, it is necessary to train men and women together for the entire life cycle. In addition to nurturing the currently required experts, investments should be made nationally to nurture the next generation of cybersecurity experts. Many countries are creating programs to train the next generation of cybersecurity leaders at the national level. Representatively, there is Korea's Best of the Best (BoB) program. Students who have completed the BoB program have won the World Hacking Competition DEFCON twice. And for such a program, it is necessary to make cybersecurity experts into a mentor pool and share the experiences and knowledge of seniors in an apprenticeship through a mentoring system.

In addition to nurturing human resources, the cybersecurity private market should be expanded, and efforts should be made to foster start-ups and large corporations. The private sector should be developed so that human resources can work creatively as well as those in the government in which they can work after receiving education and training. And these private sectors and the government should work together to protect cybersecurity and security.

6.7 Conclusion

The number of people in the MENA region who participate on the Internet is constantly increasing, and MENA countries are gradually moving toward a digital society through digital transformation. In addition, the digital society will further become a smart society. In a smart society, the development of a smart city with smart factories, smart homes, and smart mobility is inevitable. Now, the boundary line between the physical and cyber worlds is blurred, and an era in which the two worlds are united is approaching. In this new world, it is difficult to guarantee the success of the digital society unless the reliability of cybersecurity is guaranteed.

The MENA region is rapidly entering the Internet and digital society. Accordingly, many threats are occurring together. To maintain the security and peace of the MENA region from various cyberthreat actors such as cybercriminals and cyberterrorists, close cooperation among MENA countries is necessary. There is a need for a joint cybersecurity research institute, and through this, systematic assessment should be performed to proceed with developmental directions and activities. Finally, there is nothing more important in the long run than training cybersecurity talent. To strengthen cyber capabilities, it is necessary to develop and operate a cybersecurity talent training program in the MENA region throughout the life cycle. It is expected that these activities will continue to maintain cybersecurity and peace in the MENA region.

Bibliography

Aboul-Enein, S. (2017). Cybersecurity challenges in the Middle East, GenevaPapers.

Al-Tawil, K. (2001). The internet in Saudi Arabia. *Telecommunications Policy*, *25*(8), 625–634.

Bada, M., Arreguin-Toft, I., Brown, I., N. Cornish, P., Creese, S., Dutton, W. H., Goldsmith, M., et al. (2016). Cybersecurity capacity review of the United Kingdom. Global Cyber Security Capacity Centre, University of Oxford special Report, pp. 36–42.

Barclay, C. (2014). Sustainable security advantage in a changing environment: The Cybersecurity Capability Maturity Model (CM 2). In *Proceedings of the 2014 ITU Kaleidoscope Academic Conference: Living in a Converged World-Impossible without Standards?* (pp. 275–282). IEEE.

Healey, J., & Bochoven, L. V. (2012). *Nato's cyber capabilities: Yesterday, today, and tomorrow*. Atlantic Council of the United States.

Index, ITU Global Cybersecurity. (2018). https://www.itu.int/en/ITU-D/Cybersecurity

Internet usage in the Middle East. https://www.internetworldstats.com/stats5.htm

Ji-Young, K., In, L. J., & Gon, K. K. (2019). The all-purpose sword: North Korea's cyber operations and strategies. In *2019 11th International Conference on Cyber Conflict (CyCon)* (Vol. 900, pp. 1–20). IEEE.

Kim, K.-g. (2017). *State-sponsored hacker and changes in hacking techniques*.

Klaus, S. (2019). *The global competitiveness report 2019, world economic forum*. http://www3.weforum.org/docs/WEF_TheGlobalCompetitivenessReport2019.pdf

NDTAR. (2019). *National digital transformation annual report 2019*. https://ndu.gov.sa/report/ndu-annual-report-en.pdf

Oz, H., Aris, A., Levi, A., & Uluagac, A. S. (2021). A survey on ransomware: Evolution, taxonomy, and defense solutions. arXiv preprint arXiv:2102.06249

PwC. (2016). *Adjusting the lens on the economic crime in the Arab World*. http://www.pwc.com/m1/en/publications/documents/economic-crime-in-the-arabworld-2016.pdf

Resilience, Deterrence. (2017). *Defence: Building strong cybersecurity for the EU: Adopted by the European Commission on 13 September 2017/European Union*. https://eur-lex.europa.eu/legalcontent/EN/TXT

Salem, F. (2017). The Arab World Online 2017: Digital transformations and societal trends in the age of the 4th industrial revolution. Volume 3.

The National. (2012). *Cyber warfare in the Middle East is no game*. http://www.thenational.ae/business/industry-insights/technology/cyber-warfare-in-the-middleeast-is-no-game

Transforming our world: The 2030 agenda for sustainable development. https://sdgs.un.org/2030agenda

UN Broadband Commission for Digital Development. (2015). Cyber violence against women and girls: A world-wide wake-up call. http://www2.unwomen.org/~/media/headquarters/attachments/sections/library/publications/2015/cyber_violence_genderreport.pdf?v=1&d=20150924T154259

7

POLICY IMPLICATIONS

Climate Change and Violent Extremism in Securing Our Common Future

Thomas Wuchte

7.1 Introduction

7.1.1 *As the World Burns We Fight*[1]

There is a common theme that we face a point requiring a resolve to action. Yet, the related question being asked by the author is whether we are mortgaging our future by not focusing on the impact of climate change and such areas as conflict, gender-based violence, and disaffected youth who are vulnerable to violent extremism. A great, recent article questions whether, within foreign policy, the agenda is one of extinction. *As the world loses time to act, leaders are working to dominate the remains of a ruined planet. At a moment when the imperatives of survival demand unprecedented global cooperation for decarbonization, the question preoccupying many is over how many kinetic conflicts to consider.*[2]

One would hope that the better part of humanity would have come out the other side of the COVID-19 pandemic with a renewed sense of purpose – tackling such challenges as climate change, lifting poverty conditions within developing countries, solving water deficits, and forming collective approaches to the loss of natural habitat for species other than humankind. As young diplomats, many sat transfixed by the burning twin towers and today recall thinking to one another, "This is bad, but we can't overreact, or we will squander the international goodwill." The past several years have added fuel to some of the decisions we made in the responses to terrorism and COVID-19 which empowered uninterrupted "stay-at-home" time to receive excellent disinformation that fuels current disagreements in politics.

There can be hope for a future consensus as evidenced in the early 2000s. Many participated in multilateral meetings where even our most unlikely partners – countries east of Vienna for example – pledged and truly committed efforts to

DOI: 10.4324/9781003569084-8

identify the sources of these traditional terrorism threats. For this climate change nexus, it will take a concerted decision collectively to convene a process that makes the established security structures work with unexpected partners, and (perhaps) change the resource-sharing burden away from hard security to better fund the climate conditions conducive to violent extremism. The reality, since the recent resurgence of populist policies, is that there has not been political will to redirect these resources – because spending more on the underlying conditions is often outside the remit of traditional security capacity-building. Multilateralism should now focus beyond traditional threats less (state conflict, terrorism, arms control, and nonproliferation, for example) while strengthening constructive engagement on those conditions that are pressing but considered nontraditional security threats (e.g., climate change, poverty conditions, water, and loss of natural habitat).[3] These are equal peace and security concerns among countries of this ever-smaller globe.

7.2   Chapter Foundation

7.2.1   *Focus Shifting from Militarizing Foreign Policy*

Nontraditional and traditional threats together act as a Molotov cocktail. Although traditional security concerns have created, for example, a large counterterrorism architecture in recent years with the aptly called "War on Terrorism", nontraditional security concerns that are the unresolved legacies remain ever more boiling like an unwatched kettle. Given the multifaceted but softer security challenge facing us with climate change, multilateral bodies must seize the chance to breathe life back into conflict prevention and confidence-building tools, which can serve as a valuable resource and partner for regions most at risk. While the current global disagreements portray reluctance to embrace preventive diplomacy as it applies to climate change and violent extremism, there should be a forward-looking call for leadership to expand the definition of transnational and nontraditional security challenges as core work.

Returning to the nexus of these concerns and climate change, this chapter's outset takes the view that we can and should move beyond calls to understand the linkages between the effects of climate change and the risks of recruitment to violent extremism – the past 20 years are replete with evidence by a large cadre of experts and data and studies that can point to such linkages that we have had presented as the counterterrorism architecture has grown.[4] Violent extremist groups will leverage governance failures to increase the effects of climate change. How to respond is about elevating this as a threat to peace and security with a similar consensus within the United Nations (these thoughts were developed at the high-level UN General Assembly week in 2023) and cascading downwards to regional organizations and then national priorities.

7.3 Challenges Will Rise if Not Linked

7.3.1 Conflict Zones Are Most at Risk by a Warming Earth

Researchers have drawn upon measures related to climate equality to highlight correlations between discrimination and violence at the societal level, and the likelihood of conflict. Advancing a more diverse climate perspective is increasingly recognized as a key success factor for the development of more effective policies, as well as efforts for international peace and security. Studies show that, for example, women's participation in peace negotiations increases the probability of violent conflict ending. So should the participation of those most affected by extreme climate changes (Figure 7.1).

The shortage or misdirection of resources to combat climate change in security and defense forces operations affects strategies, performance, efficiency, and most importantly, the capacity to understand and respond to the needs of communities.[5] This creates a communication and protection gap, which also hinders community engagement that is vital to addressing violent extremism. Environmental action will empower undervalued local contributions to conflict prevention, peacekeeping, conflict resolution, peacebuilding and post-conflict reconstruction missions.

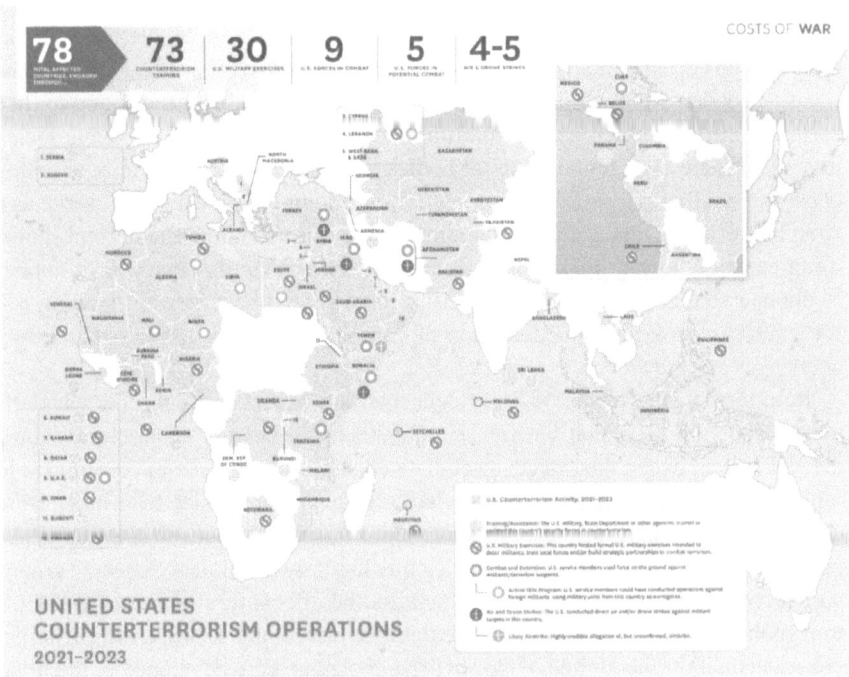

FIGURE 7.1   USA counterterrorism operations

Source: Watson Institute for International and Public Affairs (2024).

Climate change, addressed well, such as United Nations Security Council Resolution 1325 on women, peace and security, will lead further toward a recognition that these issues are deeply connected.

Later in the chapter through some examples, it will be briefly mentioned that the impact of climate change is most extreme in regions and countries that are both environmentally marginal and where governance is weakest. In many cases, these are also regions where conflict is already a high risk. Six of the top 10 countries at most risk of climate disaster are also in the top 20 countries most impacted by potential conflict or unrest.[6] Violent extremism is fueled by a deficit of humanitarian support through resources and developmental aid that support good governance. We must address the underlying conditions with local resources along with right-sized capacity-building that recognizes many now were not born at the high point post 9/11. Violent extremism as a subset of the terrorism nexus will have to change the burden sharing from hard security to a more structured distribution of time, resources, and effort.

7.4   Shifting Resources?

7.4.1   Not Gone but Risk Seen as Endemic

The author refers to a recent exchange within one article covering four observations. This is a view that underpins the basic direction of what over 20 years have wrought: an unclear future but one that has consumed many resources through the militarization of foreign policy. This article points to this sort of entropy in the international landscape of terrorism. But new challenges arise, like climate change, and the phenomenon of foreign terrorist fighters (FTFs) is not new, although it took on a new significance and magnitude over the past 20 years (Byman, 2023).

Point 1: "For an organization that once struck fear into the hearts and minds of millions of Americans after Sept. 11, 2001, and sparked a so-called global war on terror that dramatically reoriented U.S. foreign policy for two decades, al Qaeda's almost complete disappearance from both the daily news headlines and the broader foreign-policy conversation in Washington these days is remarkable."

Point 2: "According to data from the New America Foundation, jihadis have killed 107 Americans on U.S. soil since 9/11, compared with the 130 killed by right-wing terrorists."

Point 3: "To be clear, the picture is not all bad for jihadis – in Africa, new jihadi organizations are emerging, and strong groups such as al-Shabab in Somalia are flourishing – but decline is evident in most of the rest of the world."

Point 4: "With variations, this broad counterterrorism campaign began under U.S. President George W. Bush after 9/11 and continued in the Barack Obama, Donald Trump, and now Joe Biden administrations, suggesting that it has considerable staying power regardless of which party is in the White House."

Rather than asking whether Al Qaeda is relevant or not, the global counterterrorism architecture should and could shift to addressing this threat as an endemic one with maintenance of the tools already fighting terrorism, which are many, while accepting that there will be peaks and troughs in this effort. The threat is there but these episodic moments of quiet inevitably see resources shift until a new wake up. This chapter is being written amid a peak – the Hamas attack on Israel.[7] But the author generally prefers the phrase War on Terrorism without so-called – because as this article above points out that the "war" has tamped down for now many of the concerns if the New American Foundation data is accurate that more Americans were affected by domestic terrorism.

While remaining vigilant, we also need to begin to include the linkages between the effects of climate change and the risks of recruitment to a new and likely driver of violent extremism; how violent extremist groups leverage governance failures to address the effects of climate change; and how to respond, potentially developing synergies between efforts to mitigate climate change and those to build community resilience. It is not until the traditional security threats are resolved (or at least engaged in dialogue) that we may then turn, now in collaboration, to the larger problems of health crises, rising poverty, and climate change which many point to as the more strategic and long-term threats.

7.5 Broadening Violent Extremism in Terrorism to Include Climate Change

7.5.1 The Lesson of Foreign Terrorist Fighters Is We Can Work Together

For 20 years now, terrorism and its subsequent violent extremism has been about risk management – managing a risk to which our societies are particularly averse. This is, after all, the aim of terrorists – manipulating public opinions and influencing policy by instilling fear. The temptation may therefore be very high to take drastic measures, blanket restrictions. The preceding section juxtaposes the threat, as originally defined, with one more endemic.[8] How does this reflect the process since 9/11?

Governments should have taken the time to weigh options and consider long-term impact, not only immediate security benefits but broader implications on society, human rights, cohesion. Many will say they did, but violent extremism continues. There is no doubt that intelligence gathering and surveillance are necessary to fight terrorism and protect the right to life – but similarly to protect the right to life, we will now have to include climate change. The challenge is to ensure that these operations along with environmental concerns are targeted, proportionate, and even more non-discriminatory. There is already good precedent.

As an example, the international community has a very good memory about what has happened regarding associated designations for foreign terrorist fighters and shows the power that the UN Security Council can equally bear on climate change. UN Security Council Resolution 2178 (2014) and its successor, UN Security Council Resolution 2396 (2017), provided greater focus on measures to address those traveling to and then returning from and relocating foreign terrorist fighters and transnational terrorist groups. They were successful by all accounts. Both resolutions were, at that time, citing "the Islamic State in Iraq and the Levant (ISIL) also known as Da'esh, the Al-Nusrah Front (ANF) and other cells, affiliates, splinter groups or derivatives of ISIL, Al-Qaida or other terrorist groups..." (United Nations Security Council Resolution 2178, 2014)

Finally, for full context, these resolutions provided this language in UNSCR 2178: "Expressing grave concern over the acute and growing threat posed by foreign terrorist fighters, namely individuals who travel to a State other than their States of residence or nationality for the purpose of the perpetration, planning, or preparation of, or participation in, terrorist acts or the providing or receiving of terrorist training, including in connection with armed conflict, and resolving to address this threat...", and then UNSCR 2396 noted, "Recalling Resolution 2178 and the definition of foreign terrorist fighters, and expressing grave concern over the acute and growing threat posed by foreign terrorist fighters returning or relocating, particularly from conflict zones, to their countries of origin or nationality, or to third countries" (United Nations Security Council Resolution, 2396).

The author notes that, among the members of the UN Security Council, terrorism found a unifying theme – and particularly with FTFs. Russia's aggression toward Ukraine and its aftermath have shown that such a consensus is frayed now and unlikely to be replicated in a similar resolution. However, the precedent to consider FTFs a threat to peace and security found consensus and drove many changes on international travel. Despite the success of these resolutions regarding travel to-and-from conflict zones, much of this was followed by a groundswell of violent extremism attacks which included the following:

i The wave of ISIS-inspired attacks began to spread rapidly across Western Europe in the mid-2010s. ISIS-inspired attacks peaked between 2015 and 2017 (including, among others, the 2015 Charlie Hebdo shooting; 2015 Paris Bataclan attacks; 2016 Nice Bastille Day truck attack; 2016 Berlin Christmas market attack; 2017 Westminster Bridge attack; 2017 Manchester Arena bombing; 2017 Barcelona attacks).

ii The consequent far-right politics and violent extremist attacks then followed.

iii Isolated attacks continue to threaten global security. Preventing and countering violent extremism (P/CVE) is critical for each region given that, for example, according to Europol's Terrorism Situation and Trend Report 2020, of the arrests made in Europe relating to "jihadist terrorism" in 2019, in more than 70% of cases the individuals arrested were nationals of the EU country in question.

Climate change will create conditions ripe for violent extremism, and this will require new approaches. Nowadays we have fighters from recent conflict zones that are not, for example, Iraq and Syria. Which leads to the question of whether this changes the definition of FTFs? One can expect that soon we will point to this debate and say that's different from the way FTFs were defined previously regarding ISIL, Da'esh and others. Although we cannot know what the outcome of this debate will be, we should be pleased to read that we have opened a discussion that UN member states will have to come back to as threats evolve. The next definition is unlikely to be like the one set out in the above quoted resolutions. And, because it will not fully suit member state's needs or their understanding of the violent extremism issue, one will have to consider any definition vis-à-vis climate change.

7.5.2 A Ready-Made Source of Concern

The United Nations Analytical Support and Sanctions Monitoring Team noted that some 15,000 people went to fight with listed groups associated with Al Qaida in Syria and Iraq. Since 2010, these numbers were many times the size of the numbers of FTFs between 1990 and 2010. More than 80 countries, including from throughout climate-risk countries, had nationals or residents involved in the problem, including countries that have not previously faced challenges relating to Al Qaida.[9]

As noted in the end of the last section, regionally many were facing unprecedented numbers of individuals departing to join terrorist groups and/or to perpetrate acts of terrorism, including in connection with regional conflicts. Moreover, many more individuals were vulnerable to violent radicalization and recruitment as FTFs. These returnees were nurtured by violent extremist views, often exploiting beliefs and tenets as part of broader narratives built around real or perceived grievances such as ascendant climate change. Many former terrorists have now returned to their countries of nationality or residence, presenting a risk that they will further contribute to spread similar views or get involved in attacks and other terrorism-related offences. Climate change can be expected to unleash several factors that could combine these forces with displaced livelihoods and populations (Freedman, 2023).

7.6 How to Approach This Nexus

7.6.1 Collaboration and Empathy Plus Resources

Regarding counterterrorism (CT) strategies and barriers that are inevitably going to rise when arguing for inclusion of climate. The UN and regional bodies, as well as coordinated multilateral actions, will be necessary for those who share similar views. Equally, countries must be encouraged to take the lead in promoting international cooperation just like previously with the issue of foreign terrorist fighters.[10] After 20 years of overseeing collective capacity-building efforts to address post-9/11 gaps in legislation, administrative measures, and overall awareness, governments should consider collaboration – that is a true strategic partnership with climate beneficiary countries – as the better model than viewing capacity-building purely as offering aid or technical cooperation from a largely Western donor perspective (Figure 7.2).

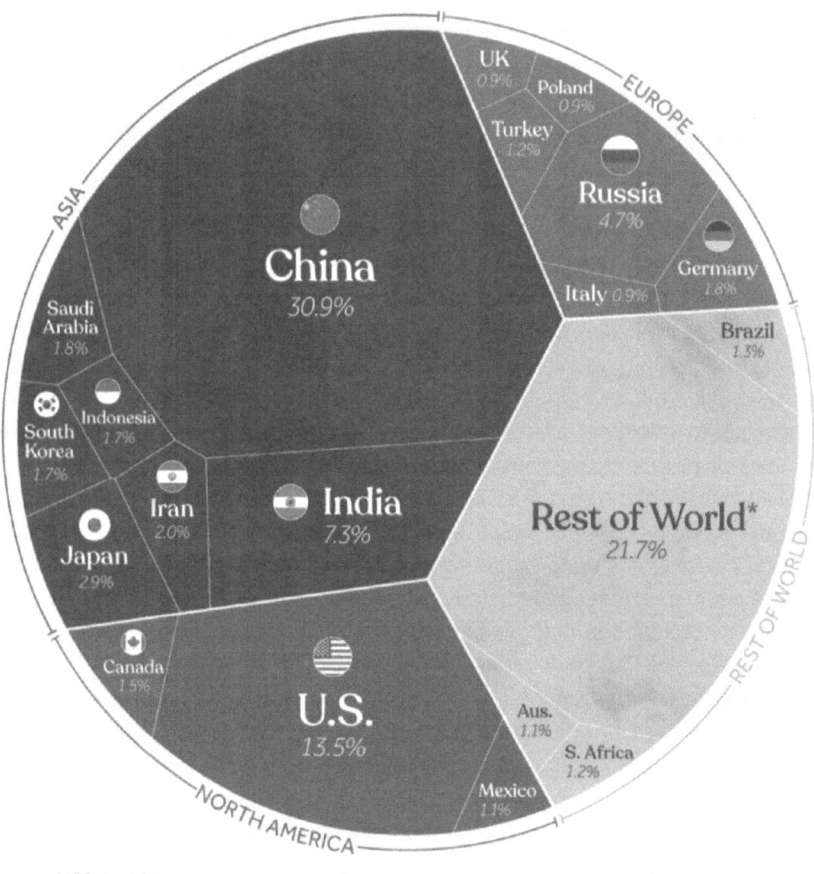

FIGURE 7.2 Global Carbon Atlas

Source: Lu (2023).

Even after 20 years of robust funding under the rubric of the War on Terrorism, do we leave anything tangible in human resource capital locally? Lots of discussions and training but going beyond cooperation to work collaboratively with partners at the earliest stage, identifying priorities and linking objectives by sharing and coordinating resources by and amongst donors – this, in essence, should be the approach of the capacity-building – including the provision of more human resources. With climate change, violent extremism can be addressed early on by taking these lessons and leading action before the effects are breeding more terrorist concerns.

The first quality which the author always emphasizes is collaboration with empathy. Several challenges exist with climate change, despite repeated calls for cooperation to adequately safeguard this as a human right, these include political challenges. On the one hand, policymakers may lack the political will or on the other hand there may be wherewithal to develop and implement measures based on the rule of law and international law decisions arising from climate summits that hardly if at all consider violent extremism yet. In addition, we see multilateral constraints: for example, security sector oversight and accountability mechanisms may be non-existent, dysfunctional, corrupt, inadequately transparent, independent, or not enforceable at all; or may impose differing standards between various agencies. There may be structural constraints, such as under-resourcing, a lack of institutional and professional capacity or a prevailing culture of institutional non-support to treat this nexus as a rising security threat equal to terrorism as traditionally defined. Inadequate training is also prevalent, as most collaboration for practitioners even today features only passing mention of regional cooperation on emerging (non-kinetic) threats, briefly touching upon human rights conventions instead of encouraging participants to integrate human rights fully into their daily work and providing examples of how to do so with climate change. All of this requires empathy for the challenges in the regional or national context. Hard-learned experience is that one must avoid unconscious bias from the values of their background but embrace the local context which one should draw from as a major outcome from the thousands of counterterrorism workshops with various regions for partnership. Can we not leverage such non-military expertise now before climate change inevitably creates conditions for violent extremism? (Farrow, 2018)

Just as in the lessons from traditional counterterrorism, the key stakeholder groups would be a) managerial-level decision-makers and senior-level practitioners – in particular heads of agencies and counterterrorism units; b) mid-level practitioners, such as climate officials (provided the resources exist to onboard such positions in countries most affected) and violent-extremist specialists who are involved in counterterrorism policymaking and implementation, as well as in the investigation, prosecution, and adjudication of counterterrorism cases; c) local and regional human rights institutions concerned with climate change, civil society organizations, and community groups; and d) parliamentarians – who propose, amend, and adopt counterterrorism legislation and scrutinize governments' behavior to ensure that, in striking a balance between protecting citizens and promoting their liberty, human rights and the rule of law are respected while addressing climate effects.

The main themes and different steps would include approaches already used in the current war on terrorism adapted for inclusion of climate change risks:

1 Understanding the complexity of a strategy with climate change, the life cycle of terrorist radicalization, the push and pull factors (structural, individual, inter-personal) that increase vulnerability and drive violent extremism, and conversely the protective factors that strengthen resilience, including the gendered and youth differences in these issues
2 Promoting the human rights at stake in a climate-change strategy as well as in traditional P/CVE
3 Explaining climate change as a policy field for any national security, requiring a multi-dimensional and multi-stakeholder approach, including both inter-agency collaboration and public–private partnerships (whole-of-government and whole-of-society); understanding national and international policy frameworks
4 Outlining the similarities, differences, and possible inter-linkages with other challenges to human rights and social cohesion, such as marginalization, disen-franchisement, intolerance, xenophobia, hate crimes, corruption, and injustice
5 Supporting the different ways in which civil society can contribute, how this needs to be context and gender and youth sensitive, and how this may be di-rectly focused on violent extremism or contribute to climate mitigation rather indirectly, including knowledge of concrete examples of civil society projects/initiatives that illustrate these efforts and can serve as an inspiration
6 Knowing where to find further reliable information, existing networks that can be joined, and support mechanisms that exist
7 Addressing gender, faith, and inter-generational issues/aspects in all groups given their crosscutting nature

In practice, European Union Advisory Mission in Iraq (EUAM Iraq), in con-junction with the Clingendael Institute, organized a dialogue on "Climate Secu-rity is National Security" in Basra, where representatives from the government, civil society, non-governmental organizations, as well as policy and thematic experts discussed the existential climate crises through the prism of national se-curity. The need for collective and integrated policy analysis and action to adapt and mitigate climate change was emphasized, as was the inclusion of climate security in all policy areas and the development of integrated and institutional responses.

The event helped to clarify and reinforce the fact that climate security is a threat multiplier and a fundamental national security imperative (The European Union Advisory Mission in Iraq, 2023). The inputs will contribute to develop policy rec-ommendations for the Iraqi government as part of the development of the new Na-tional Security Strategy (NSS). The organizers noted that climate security refers to the impact of climate crisis on peace and security. Climate change can trigger com-petition for natural resources, insecure livelihoods, and mass displacement, and thus increase the risk of social tensions and instability. It constitutes a significant threat to national security. Iraq is one of the five countries in the world worst affected by climate change. About 92% of Iraqi land is threatened by desertification, and temperatures are increasing seven times faster than the global average. (See United Nations Iraq.)

7.6.2 An Example from the Balkan Route

Primary prevention in P/CVE work, such as awareness raising, requires common terminologies and a shared understanding of local and regional factors that drove people to action. In the previous sections regarding FTF travel to Syria and Iraq, much effort has been and continues to focus on the rehabilitation and reintegration of these returnees, as processes of tertiary prevention, which require even more stable relationships between frontline practitioners and security and non-security institutions as well as between practitioners and returnees, to be able to develop the trust needed for social and functional interventions. The same will be true for those affected by climate change.

The rapid arrival of hundreds of thousands of migrants into the European Union (EU) from the Middle East, South Asia, and Africa beginning in 2015 coincided with an increase in support for anti-immigrant rhetoric and the far-right in many European countries. A substantial number of these migrants came to the EU through what became known as the "Balkan Route" a major transit land route cutting through the western Balkans. In 2016, however, the Route officially "closed," leaving many of those people attempting to reach Europe effectively stranded within the Balkans. In 2020, for example, approximately 7,000 migrants and refugees were present within the borders of just one Balkan state at any given time (Lažetić, 2021). This presence of migrants within the Balkans did not go unnoticed and, in some cases, even spurred increased activity within and mobilization among far-right actors opposed to their presence in the region.

The precarious situation of several thousand migrants who had been stuck in the Balkans attempting to reach Western Europe, coupled with the intensification of anti-immigrant campaigns, has been further exacerbated in the wake of the COVID-19 pandemic. One can expect climate change to eventually create a new surge along many routes. Because governments took some of the most stringent steps to stop the COVID-19 epidemic, the pandemic coincided with a rise in anti-immigrant sentiment worldwide, which had the impact of mainstreaming some far right views and discourse. It is estimated that about 40% of citizens believe in conspiracy theories related to migrants (Lažetić, 2021). During curfews imposed by one government in 2020, for example, migrants were restricted from leaving asylum centers regardless of the reason. While this policy was in keeping with broader measures that restricted movement even among citizens, migrants were additionally subjected to the deployment of the army to guard asylum and reception centers. Both restrictions on migrants' movement outside of the centers and the army's presence at those centers continued even after protective measures were relaxed for the rest of the population. The deployment of military resources to asylum centers was justified by their president as a means of providing "protection" to local populations. The precedent and conditions are set for a similar reaction with climate change movement.

7.7 The Inclusion of the Most Vulnerable – Climate Change

7.7.1 Addressing the Most Affected Cohorts

Having a calibrated, individual approach is especially crucial when dealing with vulnerable cohorts, especially youth. When no crime has been committed, we should be careful not to further alienate young people and push them down the wrong path through inappropriate reaction – whether denial or repression – of their climate voices. Each case must be assessed individually to establish to what extent the young person espouses narratives (not taking an odd visit to a seemingly extremist website at face value) and the reasons why. Helping vulnerable young people distance themselves from violent extremism will require varying degrees of ideological and emotional engagement. This is a difficult thing to do, which requires sensitivity and a certain degree of knowledge. Families, community members, teachers, must be able to find the resources and counsel to address these situations.

During the past 20 years in various leadership capacities addressing traditional counterterrorism, the author has seen the international community come together during times of great change and challenge. Are we developing synergies between efforts to mitigate climate change and those to build community resilience for youths? Mostly a no – I would refer to the well-recognized Stockholm International Peace Research Institute (SIPRI) and its article in June of 2023 that laments that the Security Council has yet to make climate change a standing item on its agenda – this is an overdue action (Day & Krampe, 2023). The greatest security challenges to humankind are not always traditional warfare or terrorism (though of course these remain significant considerations, and were only exacerbated by COVID-19 and the further rise of populism).

Climate change is a threat multiplier, aggravating existing inequalities and unrest, and bringing with it a vast range of unprecedented security issues which our multilateral organizations such as the UN are not able to place at the forefront of their security agendas. Multilateral institutions must therefore be further repurposed, reprioritizing their security focus toward the imminent, but they find it harder to measure threats of the future which include violent extremism arising from climate change. Multilateral organizations, starting with the UN, must reconsider their spending priorities, which primarily remain focused on traditional "hard" security issues such as military preparedness and nonproliferation, arms control, disarmament, and counterterrorism.

Although the UN Global Counter-Terrorism Strategy builds on four pillars and gives a clear understanding of practically all fields which are to be considered both when identifying and when tackling terrorism challenges, these robust plans preventing violent extremism face the competing demands of resources for other priorities which will now include climate-change effects. While these action plans hopefully will draw attention for the legislative colleagues to factor resources which can bring us forward – to turn words into action and action into climate partnership – these priorities have often been misunderstood or under-estimated by day-to-day constituency views that foreign assistance collaboration on the underlying conditions (Pillar I) and how they affect are not "priority" as the investment yet for climate change in the context of terrorism. Here the UN must play the key role in elevating climate change as a threat to peace and security.

7.8 A Way Ahead – Pillar I: Conditions Conducive to Terrorism

7.8.1 Elevating Pillar 1 to Support Climate Change

Broadening the scope of the UN's security sector reform to address the resources more fully and political will to change these underlying these conditions – known as Pillar 1 in the United Nations Climate Change Strategy – addressing the conditions conducive to the spread of terrorism. This emphasis would seek donor pledges to address as stated in UNSCR 2178: "[T]he conditions conducive to the spread of violent extremism, which can be conducive to terrorism, including by empowering youth, families, women, religious, cultural and education leaders, and all other concerned groups of civil society and adopt tailored approaches to countering recruitment to this kind of violent extremism and promoting social inclusion and cohesion" (RAN Issue Paper, 2016). Now we must add climate change.

Over the past 20 years we have come to understand that radicalization that leads to violent extremism is in many cases an individual process defined through the lens of traditional hard security with a largely kinetic approach. It is hard to understand the motives, it is hard to understand what should have been done differently by the state, by the communities, and by family members and peers. We are not far from the truth in saying that every radicalization case needs a tailor-made solution. From this perspective, one can wonder if more training as capacity-building alone on the prevention of violent extremism does not take the focus from where we really need them – focusing more on the role of the conditions conducive to terrorism that will be embodied in the consequences of climate change.

Resources are mentioned by many. Funding conflict is the short-term bet but are we willing to consider traditional security beneficiaries as either accepting burden sharing or adding climate change to their fundamental work while reallocating monies to the underlying conditions versus more securitization. This will be a rightsizing to support local communities. It takes billions, not millions, to mitigate climate change. Creating connections between initiatives to reduce climate change and increase community resilience.

With shifting of resources, cooperation and action could include the following:

- Fund, encourage, and develop networked climate change relations with and across international organizations while deemphasizing the hard security solution (essentially accepting risk), noting where guidelines, legislation, and measures might be mutually recognized or harmonized, whether regionally or sub-regionally.
- Create more sub-regional activities and tailored dialogues on the conditions conducive to terrorism built around climate change for more explicit sharing and comparing of experiences and lessons learned on implementation outcomes, including assistance that is delivered with resources and not solely as two- to three-day one-off training intervention.
- Strengthen funding for information exchanges on missions and needs assessments made by international organizations by networking among a climate change advocates at the UN, among member states and within international organizations as part of the assessments.
- When cooperating with regional and subregional organizations, consider the foremost priorities of development, economic, and security issues in an integrated or resource-priority approach as part of capacity-building – no militarized training without development aid on site.
- Undertaking measures to fulfill aspects of climate urgency must be complementary to efforts dealing with other priority development issues, including post-conflict reconstruction, and with regional security expertise for states to draw from to build climate resources on par with the architecture created to mitigate terrorism.

The final step is that political will must embrace deep multilateral perspectives and systemic support to this process. The whole is stronger than the individual and member states must again embrace multilateral work. The results sometimes take longer, but the buy-in is always better. The outcomes one would foresee could have the following impacts:

1 Practitioners and policymakers are better equipped with the knowledge to identify existing gaps and vulnerabilities in their multilateral approach to violent extremism driven by climate change, as well as adjust any structural and/or functional flaws within these institutions.
2 Practitioners have the skills to address the gaps and vulnerabilities they identify by applying international standards, legislation, and procedures when further developed that effectively integrate multilateral policymaking on climate change.
3 Practitioners are equipped with the tools to share knowledge they have acquired with fellow practitioners at the national and regional levels and to ensure that the approaches are adequately codified and/or institutionalized while allocating less resources to the militarization of foreign policy.

Focus on traditional security is not only overly prioritized with resources, but it is a dangerous distraction from future threats that are outside hard-security budgets. There is time to combat, and mitigate, these disparities; but that window is closing fast. And to do this effectively, it is not sufficient simply to shift our security focus. We must reinvigorate our international multilateral security organizations with more resources so that climate change and violent extremism do not form another driver of instability.

Notes

1 The views in this chapter are solely those of the author and do not represent the opinions of current or past organizations.
2 Drawn from Ackerman (2023).
3 At present, the trend remains bleak to make this shift. The 2023 UN Climate Change Conference demonstrated mixed constructive engagement by oil, coal and gas producers (Frost, 2023).
4 See, for example, Bourekba (2021) as well as published on this topic with the US Institute of Peace (USIP). You can find the USIP brief here which notes that the US Department of Defense has longstanding efforts on the impact of changing climate conditions on defense infrastructure and the operating environment (Burke, 2023).
5 See Corbett (2023). Taken altogether, this map's data highlights that the expansive global counterterrorism apparatus grinds ever onwards according to the Costs of War Project report: https://www.commondreams.org/news/joe-biden-war-on-terror.
6 Drawn from Side Event on the Margins of the 78th UN General Assembly (2023). In fact, one group of experts recently suggested that only a 'misreading of the state of science' could allow any doubt over the links between climate change and insecurity (Buhaug et al., 2023)
7 Linkages are quickly adapted by both international and domestic terrorism. One can expect climate change to be a convenient driver (CNN, 2023).
8 For an alternate view driven by the recent Israeli-Hamas crisis (Harmouch, 2023).
9 See Admin (2014). Though the current conflicts are not of Al-Qaida's making, it has animated supporters and mobilized reactions that they could harness. Here one can see climate change as a sentiment ripe for similar exploitation. Also see Bacon (2023).
10 This consensus will be challenging, as some of the largest carbon footprints are by countries who have yet to agree to place this climate change on the Security Council agenda for counterterrorism – e.g., China and India (Visual Capitalist, 2023).

References

Ackerman, S. (2023). US foreign policy has an extinction agenda. *The Nation*. Retrieved December 2023, from https://www.thenation.com/article/environment/climate-change-foreign-policy/

Admin. (2014). Sixteenth report of the analytical support and sanctions monitoring team, pursuant to resolution 2161. Retrieved December 2023, from https://www.security councilreport.org/atf/cf/%7B65BFCF9B-6D27-4E9C-8CD3-CF6E4FF96FF9%7D/s_2014_770.pdf

Bacon, T. (2023). The jihadist landscape amidst Israel-Hamas war: Five critical factors. International Center for Counter-Terrorism. Retrieved December 2023, from https://www.icct.nl/publication/jihadist-landscape-amidst-israel-hamas-war-five-critical-factors?trk=feed-detail_main-feed-card_feed-article-content

Bourekba, M. (2021). Climate change and violent extremism in North Africa. Barcelona Centre for International Affairs (CIDOB), 15–16. Retrieved December 2023, from https://www.cidob.org/en/publications/publication_series/project_papers/cascades/climate_change_and_violent_extremism_in_north_africa

Buhaug, H., de Coning, C., & von Uexkull, N. (2023). Should the security council engage with implications of climate change? Let's look at the scientific evidence. The Global Observatory. Retrieved December 2023, from https://theglobalobservatory.org/2023/06/security-council-climate-change-scientific-evidence/

Burke, S. (2023). Achieving climate security. https://www.usip.org/publications/2023/08/achieving-climate-security

Byman, D. (2023). Whatever happened to Al Qaeda? *Foreign Policy*. Retrieved December 6, 2023, from https://foreignpolicy.com/2023/07/31/al-qaeda-zawahiri-death-strength-decline-terrorism/ and https://www.newamerica.org/future-security/reports/terrorism-in-america/what-is-the-threat-to-the-united-states-today/

CNN. (2023). How antisemitic hate groups are using artificial intelligence in the wake of Hamas attacks. Retrieved December 2023, from https://www.cnn.com/2023/11/14/us/hamas-israel-artificial-intelligence-hate-groups-invs/index.html?trk=feed_main-feed-card_feed-article-content/

Corbett, J. (2023). 78-country map rebuffs claim that US 'not at war'. *Common Dreams*. Retrieved December 2023, from https://www.commondreams.org/news/joe-biden-war-on-terror

Day, A., & Krampe, F. (2023). Beyond the UN security council: Can the UN general assembly tackle the climate–security challenge? Stockholm International Peace Research Institute. Retrieved December 2023, from https://www.sipri.org/commentary/essay/2023/beyond-un-security-council-can-un-general-assembly-tackle-climate-security-challenge

Farrow, R. (2018). *War on peace – The end of diplomacy and the decline of American influence* (13p). W.W. Norton & Company, Inc.

Freedman, A. (2023). *COP28 has high stakes for planet as climate warms, extreme weather surges*. Axios. https://www.axios.com/2023/11/29/cop28-global-warming-high-stakes

Frost, R. (2023). Record number of fossil fuel lobbyists allowed to attend COP28 climate talks, campaigners say. *Euronews*. Retrieved December from https://www.euronews.com/green/2023/12/05/record-number-of-fossil-fuel-lobbyists-granted-access-cop28-climate-talks-campaigners-say.

Harmouch, S. (2023). Al-Qaeda: A defeated threat? Think again. War on the Rocks. Retrieved December 2023, from https://warontherocks.com/2023/11/al-qaeda-a-defeated-threat-think-again/

Lažetić, M. (2021). Migration, extremism, & dangerous blame games. Resolve Network. Retrieved December 2023, from https://www.resolvenet.org/system/files/2021-11/RSVE_WB_Report_MigrationExtremismDangerousBlame_LazeticNov.2021_0.pdf

Lu, M. (2023). Visualizing all the world's carbon emissions by country. Retrieved October 10, 2024 from https://www.visualcapitalist.com/carbon-emissions-by-country-2022/

RAN Issue Paper. (2016). The root causes of violent extremism. RAN Center of Excellence. Retrieved December from chrome-extension://efaidnbmnnnibpcajpcglclefindmkaj/https://home-affairs.ec.europa.eu/system/files/2021-05/ran_collection-approaches_and_practices_en.pdf

Side Event on the Margins of the 78th UN General Assembly. (2023). Climate change and violent extremism: Causes, consequences and solution.

The European Union Advisory Mission in Iraq. (2023, November 27). EUAM Iraq: Dialogue on the impact of climate change to national security. https://www.euam-iraq.eu/en/news/189/euam-iraq-organised-a-dialogue-on-the-impact-of-climate-change-to-national-security

United Nations Security Council Resolution 2178. (2014). Retrieved December 6, 2023, from https://documents-dds-ny.un.org/doc/UNDOC/GEN/N14/547/98/PDF/N1454798.pdf?OpenElement

United Nations Security Council Resolution 2396. (2017). Retrieved December 6, 2023, from https://documents-dds-ny.un.org/doc/UNDOC/GEN/N17/460/25/PDF/N1746025.pdf?OpenElement

Visual Capitalist. (2023). Visualizing all the world's carbon emissions by country. Retrieved December 2023, from https://www.visualcapitalist.com/carbon-emissions-by-country-2022/

Watson Institute for International and Public Affairs. (2024). United States Counterterrorism Operations under the Biden Administration 2021–2023. Retrieved October 15, 2024 from https://watson.brown.edu/costsofwar/papers/2023/USCounterterrorismOperations

8

RECOVERY STRATEGY

The Efforts of the East Timor Government in Resolving Crisis

Any Rufaedah

8.1 Introduction

East Timor is a country with a long journey of independence and peace. The country was colonized by Portugal – and partially by Dutch – for 273 years from 1702 to 1975 (Chaobang, n.d.; Svoboda & Davey, 2013). From 1945 to 1948, Japan invaded the country, resulting in deaths of about 60,000 Timor Leste. After Portuguese colonization, Indonesia under the order of president Suharto, occupied the country for 24 years from 1975 to 1999. Reports presented different estimates, from more than 100,000 to nearly 200,000, of people killed or died from famine and diseases during Indonesian occupation (Asia Foundation, 2017; Svoboda & Davey, 2013). The country just achieved its total independence in 2002 after a long process and intervention of multiple parties, including the United Nations and its neighboring country, Australia.

East Timor, which has the official name Democratic Republic of Timor-Leste and is commonly called Timor-Leste, has 13 municipalities inhabited by approximately 1,329,680 people (Statistics Timor-Leste, 2020; Worldometer, 2020). The people of East Timor were led by two presidents from 1975–1978 and four presidents after their independence. Two presidents, Vicente Guterres and Fernando de Araújo, served as acting presidents in 2008, replacing José Manuel Ramos-Horta, who was injured in an attack at his home (Goulart, 2008; Interviews: Fernando "Lasama" de Araújo, n.d.). The attack was an indicator that security issues and political rivalry were still quite high at that time.

East Timor faced a crisis in the 1970s, when Portugal gave the people of East Timor their right to hold independence. Following the independence agenda, political parties were created and ran for a different agenda. *Frente Revolucionária de Timor–Leste Independente* (Revolutionary Front for an Independent East Timor/

DOI: 10.4324/9781003569084-9

FRETILIN), which garnered support from a majority of Timorese and promoted Marxism-Leninism ideology, struggled for national independence. *União Democratica Timorense* (Timorese Democratic Union/UDT) persisted with a connection with Portugal, and another party, *Associação Popular Democrática de Timor* (Popular Democratic Association of Timor/APODETI) built a coalition with the Indonesian government (Rufaedah, 2020). Even though APODETI had a different affiliation in the beginning, it then supported UDT (Svoboda & Davey, 2013).

The differences in political ideology and interest dragged Timorese to a clash. It became worse when the Indonesian military invaded the country. On December 7, 1975, Indonesian troops launched a bombardment of the capital city of East Timor, Dili, and targeted the second largest East Timorese city, Baucau, on December 10, 1975 (History.com Editors, 2019). Another deadly event was the November 12, 1991, Santa Cruz massacre, which killed more than 250 Timorese who were gathering in Dili Santa Cruz cemetery for a march agenda (Fincher, 2018).

Following the fall of Indonesian president Suharto and pressure from a multinational United Nations force, Indonesian militias left East Timor in 1999, while Timorese continued to struggle for their total independence. Through the supervision of the UN Transitional Administration in East Timor (UNTAET) for about two years, Timorese held their independence on May 20, 2002. They elected Xanana Gusmão, the former commander in chief of FALINTIL, a military wing of FRETILIN, as the 2002–2007 president.

However, the conflict did not meet its end yet. Four years after independence, a clash emerged between people from east regions and the west who served in military and police offices. It was triggered by a view as "true fighters" of independence. The *Lorosae* (easterners) considered themselves the true fighters compared to the *Loromonu* people (westerners) (Rufaedah, 2020; Trindade & Castro, 2007). The clash brought the dismissal of approximately 600 soldiers from East Timor Defense Force (FALINTIL-FDTL/F-FTDL/*Forças Armadas de Libertação Nácional de Timor-Leste*) and later led to open conflict from 2006–2007 (Trindade & Castro, 2007).

This chapter will specifically discuss this Loromonu–Lorosae crisis. The end of the chapter discusses initiatives from the government and civil society organizations (CSOs) in handling conflict and provides an update on current security issues in East Timor.

8.2 Loromonu–Lorosae: Factors behind the Conflict

The Loromonu–Lorosae conflict took place from April to late May 2006, four years after East Timor's formal independence in 2002. The tension started with a petition from Falintil-Timor Leste Defence Force (F-FTDL) officers complaining of alleged discrimination in military and police bodies. The petition was sent on January 9, 2006, and received by President Gusmão two days later, on January 11. Unfortunately, the president and related authorities of East Timor did not send any response until February 1 (Refugee Review Tribunal Australia, 2007).

According to the Refugee Review Tribunal Australia's report (2007), following the unacknowledged petition, 418 petition senders, who were later known as petitioners, held a march at the presidential palace. The situation was getting worse as the government took an extreme decision in resolving the issue. In mid-March 595 military officers, consisting of petitioners and about 200 officers with work discipline issues, were dismissed.

The dismissal was received with protests and negotiations, and eventually brought the country to open violence in late April (25 and 28) to May (8, 23, 24, 25). The conflict was not single but multi-layered and involved former military officers, active military officers (F-FDTL), Policia Nacional de Timor-Leste (PNTL) officers, armed civilians, and the minister of interior. According to Kammen's study (2010), the conflicts that erupted on May 23 and 25 involved former commanders of the military police and F-FDTL, between armed civilians supported by the minister of interior and F-FDTL headquarters, and between the national police and F-FDTL. It also dragged in President Gusmão (associated with the west, opposing Fretilin), and F-FDTL, (associated with the East; Niner, 2008).

The clashes reportedly killed 38 people and caused a huge amount of damage. About 1,000 houses were burned and approximately 175 thousand people left their homes to seek refuge – reports showed different numbers. On the political side, the opposition coalition forced Prime Minister Mari Alkatiri to resign from his position and brought Foreign Minister José Manuel Ramos-Horta to replace him. The petition was originally addressed to President Gusmão; however, it could not force Gusmão to resign since he had turned over the petition issue to Alkatiri.

Following the conflicts, scholars conducted studies to understand the Loromonu and Lorosae more deeply in order to find the root cause of the conflicts. Trindade and Castro's study stated that *Loromonu* referred to western municipalities of East Timor, including Bobonaro, Covalima, Oecussi, Liquica, Ermera, Aileu, Ainaro, Mantuto, and Manufahi municipalities, and *Lorosae* referred to the eastern region that includes Baucau, Viqueque, and Lautem. The Loromonu were also called "Kaladi," and the Lorosae were called "Firaku." During the conflict in 2016, people commonly called Firaku "Iraq" and Kaladi "America" to associate Firaku with "terrorists" that existed in Iraq, and America was the opponent of Iraq (Kammen, 2010).

A historical study conducted by Kammen (2010) found that the terms Kaladi and Firaku originally went back to the Portuguese colonial era. There were at least three explanations describing the original meaning of Kaladi and Firaku. First, Kaladi – which was "calado" in Portuguese – was used in reference the people from the western region who were characterictly slow, quiet, and taciturn. In contrast to *calado*, Firaku (*vira o cu* in Portuguese) referred to people from the east who possessed characteristics of being temperamental and stubborn.

The second explanation was not related to characteristics or attitudes, and it was said not to come from Portuguese but from local words. Firaku was explained to come from Makassar local language: *fi,* which meant "we/us," and *raku,* which meant "relatives," while Kaladi came from a Malay/Tetum word which referred to a kind of taro growing in mountainous areas (Duarte, 1992, in Kammen, 2010). The third cited Portuguese anthropologist Paulo Castro Seixas in Trindade and Castro (2007); Kammen explained that the term Firaku meant "our comrades" in the Makasae language. The term has been adapted to "Tetum," which meant "people living in the (north)eastern mountains." Meanwhile, Kaladi was an adapted word from Mambai to Tetum, which referred to "mountainous people of the west."

Those explanations were not quite satisfactory for Kammen. Therefore, in his paper, Kammen presents historical research which helps readers to find robust explanations about the terms. The research shows that Kaladi and Firaku appeared in different eras. "Caladas" appeared first in 1720, with a meaning that referred to Indigenous people who lived out of Lifau, not in the town. However, that meaning was not the only one. Other than that, "caladas/callades" pointed to people in the upland and those who refused to acknowledge colonial masters. In Tetum, the word "caladi" meant "yam," which might refer to the food that was eaten by those who lived in the mountains (De Matos, 1974, in Kammen, 2010). In the mid-18th century, the term "firaco" appeared. Scholars suggested the term was from Makassae or Portuguese, in which it referred to politically weak polities and clans.

Jakarta militias suggested that the country be divided into east and west, with western districts (Loromonu) kept under Indonesian authority. The issue then expanded to pro-independence vs. pro-Indonesia and east vs. west. To solve the issue, the United Nations, under a request from the Indonesian president B.J. Habibie, held a vote to determine the aspirations of the Timorese on their independence. More than 78% of Timorese rejected Indonesia's offer to be a "special autonomy province," and the rest chose to remain under Indonesian administration. Although the number of people who preferred to be independent was much higher, bringing over 20% of the people who preferred to be part of Indonesia to engage in a new East Timor government was a hard challenge. It later became an issue when the number of pro-Jakarta veterans who served in the police department was considered too high.

Following the referendum result in 1999, political elites soon prepared for the election that would be held in 2001. According to Kammen's study, the tension between Loromonu/kaladi and Lorosae/firaku arose again in this period, following competition among political leaders/parties to gain voters from west and east. Other than that, the Loromonu vs. Lorosae issue emerged in the security sector, when the Falintil elites had different views in determining the leadership and form of new East Timor's defense forces (Kammen, 2010). The issue in the security sector continued till at least 2006 and became a factor which led to the 2006 crisis.

Kammen (2010) highlighted three factors triggering the east–west tension. First, an imbalanced proportion of personnel who served in the security body. A large number of former Indonesian police (POLRI) – Hood's study (2006) stated that more than 350 former POLRI were recruited in early 2000 – were signed in the new East Timor police department, Policia Nacional de Timor-Leste (PNTL). It then grew jealous of former Falintil fighters and unrecruited candidates. On the side of defense force, FALINTIL-Forças de Defesa de Timor-Leste (F-FDTL), the composition in its battalion was imbalance: Battalion I was dominated by eastern districts people and Battalion II was dominated by former fighters from the west.

Other than the formation, the foundation of the police and defense institutions were considered weak. Hood (2006) found that the United Nations Transitional Administration in East Timor, the UN body which was responsible in establishing police and military departments, did not apply or develop doctrines and strategies which would strengthen the institutions. Hood added, UNTAET failed to engage with Timor-Leste's political leaders during the establishment of PNTL. UNTAET, which was continued by UNMISET, was considered successful in providing police personnel, with recruited about 3,000 personnel in May 2004, but failed to lay the institutional foundation.

A second factor was an economic issue. One of the factors was unevenness of civil services, which was that about three-quarters of civil services, the UN, and non-governmental organizations (NGOs) were centralized in Dili (Kammen, 2010). That centralization accelerated reconstruction in Dili but slowed down the agrarian sector on the other side. The situation caused fast population growth in Dili, which led to high competition and the rapid growth of informal sectors. Trindade and Castro (2007) added that three districts in the east – Baucau, Viqueque, and Lospalos – had better soil, which made people in the east have better nutrition than people from western regions.

The third factor was rivalry among political elites. Even though Fretilin was a solid party when it was working for independence, in fact, its elites were not always working in the same direction. Xanana Gusmão, the former leader of Fretilin's military wing, Falintil, refused Fretilin's support of his effort to run in the first presidential election in 2002. Other than that, Fretilin's political competitor, Democratic Party (PD)-Social Democratic Party (PSD)-*Associação Social-Democrata Timorense*/Timorese National Democratic Association (ASDT) coalition, which dominated constituents in western districts, politically divided the Timorese into eastern and western.

The analysis does make sense. If we look at the political journey of East Timor, it was full of tension. In 2002, Gusmão, who is a former prominent figure in the biggest political party Fretilin, ran for presidential position as an independent candidate with endorsement from nine political parties outside of Fretilin. When he served as a president, he governed East Timor with his rival Mari Alkatiri as a prime minister. In 2006, Alkatiri faced pressure to resign and was replaced by Ramos-Horta, the ally of Gusmão. In the next election in 2007, Ramos-Horta ran for the presidential seat and he was shot in 2008 during his service as the second Timorese president.

Trindade and Castro (2007) added the gap in education as a trigger factor, in which residents from the east had a higher percentage of literacy than people from the western region. It meant that access to jobs was easier for easterners than for westerners. The higher gap in accessibility, which then affected economic welfare, eventually fueled jealousy and hatred that led to open violence. Trindade and Castro (2007) also highlighted the lack of progress in defining national identity and finding a formation of the state as possible contributing factors. National identity was assumed to develop by itself, and on the other side, the new East Timor adopted western systems and values without enough discussion involving all states' representatives. As a result, a lack of connection between society and government occurred.

An emerging question about the conflict is the ethnic factor: Is the conflict triggered by an ethnic issue? Seixas (in Trindade & Castro, 2007) explained that the Lorosae associated with the origin of the Timor population – the Lorosae people are Papuan/Melanesian population who migrated to the eastern half of Timor – and the Loromonu are Malayan/Indonesian population who lived in western regions. According to this explanation, the 2006 conflict involved two ethnic groups. However, scholars did not conclude that it was an ethnic-based conflict. The weakness of the national identity and political cleavage are more dominant in triggering the conflict.

Gusmão instead called the crisis a political crisis. In his 2011 speech at Johns Hopkin University, Maryland, he explicitly mentioned a "political crisis" in 2006 and was aware of a need to "grow politically" (Gusmão, 2006):

> In 2006, we had a serious political crisis that caused an atmosphere of insecurity in the Country, and various other problems that eventually led to confrontations between the Police and the Military, resulting in hundreds of thousands of internally displaced people and countless damage to the State. From these crises, we learned our first major lesson: we urgently needed to learn to deal with the fragility of our State, which resided in the inability to address the root causes of problems, resulting in a trend to avoid problems rather than seeking proper solutions. We also needed to grow politically, that is, to impose a political will within State institutions to cooperate among themselves in the search for solutions, rather than focusing on the political dimensions of every situation and, in doing so, losing the judgement required to handle and solve crises.

Studies on Timor-Leste (e.g., Trindade and Castro, 2007; Svoboda and Davey, 2013) show that the administration which prepared independence did not put in enough effort to build the foundation of the country. The transition process focused on administrative matters rather than dialog with the people. Some actors who were in charge of the administrative process, such as Xanana Gusmão, were even busy preparing their political agenda for the 2001 presidential election. The higher involvement of the United Nations in the pre-independence period compared to civil society organizations also considerably contributed to the crisis. The UN even took a crucial role in positioning police officers in the new police department, PNTL (Svoboda & Davey, 2013).

The 2006 crisis brought East Timor to a prolonged security and humanitarian problem. Even though open clashes did not occur anymore, petitioners remained to fight against the government. Under the lead of Major Alfredo Reinado, the petitioners, who were later called the "rebel group," continued their mission. Operating from the hills, the group launched threats, including a February 11, 2008, assassination attempt targeting president Ramos-Horta at his home. Prime minister Gusmão, who tried to reach Ramos-Horta's house after receiving information about the attack, was repeatedly shot on his trip (Niner, 2008). Other violent acts from various groups, including martial arts groups (MAG) and gangs (Myrttinen, 2008) kept controlling the country. In 2008, violence which burned down over 400 houses took place in Baucau city (der Auweraert, 2012).

In terms of humanitarian matters, the crisis managed to plant fear in many Timorese, as well as to exhaust the government and international communities. The International Crisis Group's report (2008) notes that approximately 30,000 displaced people decided to stay in camps, and 70,000 others were with families and friends in Dili or other districts because of fear from violence by their neighbors. This was indeed not the only reason causing internally displaced persons to keep living in camps – other reasons are discussed in the next part – however, it was considered a main factor.

8.3 How Multiple Entities Handled the Conflict

At least three actors were involved in efforts to overcome the 2006 cleavage in East Timor: the government, the UN and international entities, and Timorese non-governmental entities. As a "newborn" country, East Timor needed UN assistance and international support to resolve the problems. Nonetheless, as an established country, the government of East Timor itself had to take a crucial role, in particular in making decisions and approving proposed regulations. This section will discuss the role taken by the government of East Timor in particular, and include the assistance of UN and international entities related to the crisis.

The efforts to handle the cleavage were technically committed before the 2006 open violence. The government had held dialog with petitioners, both with petitioners' vocal point Salsinha and the groups. The United Nations Independent Special Commission of Inquiry for Timor-Leste, well known as UN Commission of Inquiry (2006), recorded that President Gusmão held a dialog with 400 petitioners and requested them to return to barracks. To convince the petitioners, the president guaranteed not to investigate them for issuing the petition. Nevertheless, those efforts were not successful to halt the anger of the petitioners and kept dragging the country to deadly unrest in April to May.

In addition, the unrest forced Prime Minister Mari Alkatiri to resign from his position along with Minister of Defense Roque Rodrigues and Minister of Interior Rogerio Lobato, who were responsible for distributing weapons to protestors (Shiosaki, 2017). Before his resignation on June 26, 2006, prime minister Alkatiri called for Australia's assistance in security matters, and it led to creation of the international stabilization force, an Australian-led force which was deployed from May 2006 to November 2012 (Svoboda & Davey, 2013), as well as called Portugal, Malaysia, and New Zealand (International Crisis Group, 2006).

The government, via the minister of foreign affairs, also requested the United Nations to establish a special body which would work to investigate the unrest. The UN responded to the request by creating the Independent Special Commission of Inquiry for Timor-Leste. In an October 2006 report, the Commission briefly described the government's request and its functions:

> The Independent Special Commission of Inquiry for Timor-Leste was established under the auspices of the United Nations High Commissioner for Human Rights following an invitation from the then Minister for Foreign Affairs of Timor-Leste to the Secretary-General to establish such a body. Its mandate was to establish the facts and circumstances relevant to incidents that took place on 28 and 29 April and 23, 24 and 25 May and related events or issues that contributed to the crisis, clarify responsibility for those events and recommend measures of accountability for crimes and serious violations of human rights allegedly committed during the mandated period.
>
> (United Nations, 2006)

Svoboda and Davey (2013) stated that in 2006, the UN mission was about to finish, and the international aid was switched to reconstruction and development programs. The crisis and the assistance needed by the government put the UN in a "no choice situation" but extended its mission. With the extended mission, the UN was recorded to have established five missions which operated in East Timor: United Nations Mission in East Timor (UNAMET, June 1999–October 1999), United Nations Transitional Administration in East Timor (UNTAET, October 1999–May 2002), United Nations Transitional Administration in East Timor (UNMISET, May 2002–May 2005), United Nations Office in Timor-Leste (UNOTIL, May 2005–August 2006), and United Nations Integrated Mission in Timor-Leste (UNMIT, August 2006–December 2012) (Svoboda & Davey, 2013). UNMIT was specifically established to assist East Timor in restoring and maintaining the security sector, including public security, PNTL, and executing a review on the security sector (Wilson, 2010).

In humanitarian issues, the government of East Timor, through the Ministry of Labour and Community Reinsertion (MTRC) and with assistance from International Organization for Migration (IOM), created the Humanitarian Coordination Group (Svoboda & Davey, 2013). In terms of financial support, East Timor received aid from UN Central Emergency Fund (CERF) and UN Office for the Coordination of Humanitarian Affairs (OCHA) (Margesson and Vaughn, 2009, in Svoboda & Davey, 2013).

The major subject handled by the government was IDPs living in camps –
as previously mentioned, an estimated 30,000 IDPs kept living in camps until
2008. Besides providing tents, the government and international agencies provided free food and basic needs (der Auweraert, 2012). Nonetheless, the facilities provided led to unpredictable negative consequences. International Crisis
Group (2008) found that the facilities attracted non-IDPs residents to come to
Dili camps on purpose to access the same provisions as well as for economic
opportunities in Dili. Other issues were the emergence of individuals who resold
free food from the government (International Crisis Group, 2008) and a complaint from IDPs who lived with relatives and friends for not receiving provisions (der Auweraert, 2012).

In December 2007, the government launched a future-oriented National Recovery Strategy (NRS) named *Hamutuk Hari'i Futuru* (Together Building the Future).
The strategy contained five pillars: together building homes, together building
protection, together building stability, together building social economy, together
building confidence/trust (Wallis, 2013a). The first strategy pillar was implemented
by returning IDPs to their homes. However, it was not easy for the government
to rebuild residents' houses. Der Auweraert (2012) noted that 3,500 destroyed or
damaged houses remained unbuilt till the end of 2008.

One of the interesting items in this NRS was a cash payment for certain groups.
The cash payment strategy was afforded for veterans who participated in resistance during the Indonesian occupation, families of veterans, and petitioners. The
veterans (former Falintil guerilla militias who fought under command of Gusmão)
were divided into three pension recipient groups: those who participated in resistance at least for eight years (Special Subsistence Pension), those who participated
for at least 15 years (Special Retirement Pension), and spouses/orphans/siblings
of veterans (Survivor Pension). The first group received cash in the range of $276
to $345 per month. The second group received between $460 and $575 per month,
and the third group received $230 to $287.50 per month. Those amounts were
applicable in 2009/2010 (Statute of the National Liberation Combatants, 2009, in
Wallis, 2013b).

Nonetheless, these categories triggered a complaint from unqualified former
fighters. In consequence, the government created a cash payment for fighters
who were involved in the resistance for four to seven years. They received a
one-off cash payment in 2019 with an amount of $1,380 (Statute of the National
Liberation Combatants, 2009, in Wallis, 2013). For the scheme, the East Timor
government reportedly spent $18.8 million in 2008, $15 million in 2009, and
$45.4 million in 2010 (MSS, 2010, in Wallis, 2010), while for the petitioners,
the government spent about $8,500 compensation for each person (International
Crisis Group, 2009).

The NRS eventually slowed down clashes in East Timor. However, the pension facilities for former pro-resistance militias alone have potentially created an

implicit division within Timorese. How former pro-Indonesia militias accept the fact of not receiving the same facilities is questioned. The government's strategy, which ran under former Falintil's leader Xanana Gusmão, can also be interpreted as a remuneration for his men. It appears more reasonable since Gusmão held power by serving as the first president from 2002–2007 and prime minister after winning the 2007 election, while not all his men earned good positions in governmental bodies. Another possible explanation behind the scheme is a political interest to persist or increase support from former Falintil militias, who were part of Fretilin political party which at that time opposed the ruling Gusmão government.

8.4 Current Security Issues in East Timor

After undergoing a long journey, what is the current security condition of East Timor? In an effort to update the current condition, I interviewed an expert and Belun staff who have worked on peace-building in Timor-Leste. Belun, which was established in 2004, is one of prominent NGOs working on the issue. Its work is based on three pillars: conflict prevention, community capacity development, research and advocacy. The first pillar is implemented with monitoring of violent conflict, understanding the root cause of conflict, planned coordinated interventions, policy making, monitoring, and evaluation. The second pillar focuses on community empowerment, and the third pillar focuses on data collection and analysis of the conflict and community issues as basic material to advocate policy change (Belun, 2019).

In terms of conflict, Belun worked on the Early Warning Early Response (EWER) program that has been implemented in two phases since 2016: 2008–2016 and 2018-present. In the first phase, Belun covered all municipalities (13) of East Timor with 43 administrative posts (sub-districts). In the second phase, it covers seven municipalities in total, with the support from the Women, Peace, and Security program of UN Women, DAP-DFAT Australia, GIZ Germany, g7+, and UNDP (situation review February–March 2020). The municipalities in the second phase were selected based on the number of incidents.

The program monitored and analyzed incidents of conflict in the administrative post (sub-district) level. To maintain sustainability of the program at a community level, Belun created community-based groups called Local Conflict Prevention Response Networks. The group involved local authority, police, youth, local NGOs, and other local stakeholders in a sub-district level as members. Each group was led by a volunteer called a "monitor." Since 2008, 43 groups have been established (Rufaedah, 2020).

Led by a monitor, group members collected conflict-related issues in their sub-district area. The findings were then sent to a coordinator who worked in Belun offices, and from the findings, the coordinator created a two-monthly report called "situation review." The situation reviews included numbers of incidents and basic information of incidents, including location, the instrument used in the incident, victims, driving factors, impacts, what Belun and the community have done within two months' work. Other than physical activity, Belun provided online incident reports that can be accessed by everyone. The report covered detailed information about the incidents, including location, date and time, the individuals involved in the accidents, and chronology of the incidents (Atres.belun.tl.).

In its strategic plan 2019–2023, Belun stated that the system has been recognized as one of the most developed early warning systems in the world. At least three countries – Myanmar, the Philippines, and Nepal – had learned the success story of the program in order to replicate the program (Rufaedah, 2020). In order to obtain maximum impact of its works, Belun shared reports and publications to the government, police, and military by in person communication or its open-access website. In the report, Belun provided recommendations and assistance for the government in implementing policies (Belun Strategic Plan, 2019–2023).

According to the Belun staff, the highest incidents at the current time are domestic violence and fighting between martial arts groups, while the ethnicity-related incidents do not exist anymore (Rufaedah, 2020). One expert interviewed made a similar statement, that ethnic-based conflict does not appear (Rufaedah, 2020). The findings indicate that the 2006 clash between the Loromonu and the Lorosae has been resolved well.

Another question that emerged is the threat of Islamic extremists against East Timor. As Indonesia's neighboring country, East Timor has a high possibility to be a targeted country, besides its status as a Catholic majority country. Nonetheless, there were no Islamic terrorism incidents reported. On May 24, 2018, 11 days after the suicide bombings in three churches in Surabaya, Indonesia, the Union of Catholic Asian News reported a warning from police on potential attacks by Islamic extremists targeting churches and bishops in Timor-Leste. Fortunately, there were no terrorist occurrences reported.

Bibliography

Asia Foundation. (2017). The state of conflict and violence in Asia: Timor-Leste. *Asia Foundation.* https://asiafoundation.org/wp-content/uploads/2017/12/Timor-Leste-State-ofConflictandViolence_revised.pdf

BBC Monitoring. (2018, February 26). East Timor country profile. *BBC* [British Broadcasting Corporation]. https://www.bbc.com/news/world-asia-pacific-14919009

Belo, J., & Sainbury, M. (2018, May 24). Terrorist fears spread to Timor-Leste as bishop threatened. *UCA News.* https://www.ucanews.com/news/terrorist-fears-spread-to-timor-leste-as-bishop-threatened/82396

Belun. (2019, March). *Strategic directions 2019–2023.*

Belun. (2020, March). *Situation review February-March 2020* [Report].

Chaobang, A. (n.d.). How well has the causality of the conflict in East Timor been reflected in its UN peacebuilding experience? *United Nations Peace and Progress, 1*(1), 33–46.

der Auweraert, P. V. (2012). Dealing with the 2006 internal displacement crisis in Timor-Leste: Between reparations and humanitarian policymaking. International Center for Transitional Justice (ICTJ) and Brookings-LSE Project on Internal Displacement.

Fincher, M. (2018, November 8). Santa Cruz massacre: Timor-Leste's democratic transition 27 years later. *Democracy Speaks*. https://www.democracyspeaks.org/blog/santa-cruz-massacre-timor-leste%E2%80%99s-democratic-transition-27-years-later

Goulart, G. (2008, February 15). East Timor declares state of emergency. *Associated Press*. https://web.archive.org/web/20080215131831/http://ap.google.com/article/ALeqM5iBwRshgYrpyGWdo136kysipYNxgAD8UOH5VO0

Gusmão, K. R. X. (2011, February 24). Goodbye conflict welcome development. [Speech text]. *Xanana Gusmao*. https://www.xananagusmao.org/goodbye-conflict-welcome-development/

Gusmão, X. (2006, April 10). *Building peace and development in East Timor* [Speech transcript]. Johns Hopkins University. https://www.exampleurl.com

History.com Editors. (2019, December 3). Indonesia invades East Timor. https://www.history.com/this-day-in-history/indonesia-invades-east-timor

Hood, L. (2006). Missed opportunities: The United nations, police service and defence force development in Timor-Leste, 1999–2004. *Civil Wars*, *8*(2), 143–162. https://doi.org/10.1080/13698240600877270

Independent Special Commission of Inquiry for Timor-Leste. (2006). *Report of the United Nations* [Report].

International Crisis Group. (2006). *Resolving Timor-Leste's crisis* [Report: Asia Report N 120, 10 October 2006]. https://www.crisisgroup.org/asia/south-east-asia/timor-leste/resolving-timor-leste-s-crisis

International Crisis Group. (2008, March 31). *Timor-Leste's displacement crisis*. International Crisis Group. https://www.crisisgroup.org/asia/south-east-asia/timor-leste/timor-leste-s-displacement-crisis

International Crisis Group. (2009). *Timor-Leste: No time for complacency* [Report: Asia Briefing N 87]. International Crisis Group. https://www.crisisgroup.org/asia/south-east-asia/timor-leste/timor-leste-no-time-complacency

Interviews: Fernando "Lasama" de Araújo. (n.d.). *The Freedom Collection*. http://www.freedomcollection.org/interviews/fernando_quotlasamaquot_de_arajo/

Kammen, D. (2010). Subordinating Timor: Central authority and the origins of communal identities in East Timor. *Bijdragen tot de Taal-, Land- en Volkenkunde*, *166*(2/3), 244–269.

Myrttinen, H. (2008, April 1). Timor Leste — A kaleidoscope of conflicts. Watch Indonesia! https://www.watchindonesia.de/1222/timor-leste-kaleidoscope-of-conflicts?lang=en

Niner, S. (2008, February 18). Major Alfredo Alves Reinado: Cycles of torture, pain, violence. *APSNet Policy Forum*. https://nautilus.org/apsnet/major-alfredo-alves-reinado-cycles-of-torture-pain-violence/

Porter, D., & Rab, H. (2010). Timor-Leste's recovery from the 2006 crisis: Some lessons. The World Bank.

Refugee Review Tribunal [RRT] Australia. (2007, March 2). *RRT research response* [Report].

Rufaedah, A. (2020, December 13). Personal interview.

Shiosaki, E. (2017). "We have resisted, now we must build": Regionalism and nation-building in Timor-Leste. *Journal of Southeast Asian Studies*, *48*(1), 53–70. https://doi.org/10.1017/S0022463116000173

Statistics Timor-Leste. (2020). *Municipality in figure*. General Directorate of Statistics. https://www.statistics.gov.tl/category/survey-indicators/timor-leste-in-figures/municipality-in-figure/#

Svoboda, E., & Davey, E. (2013). *The search for common ground: Police, protection, and coordination in Timor-Leste*. Humanitarian Policy Group.

Trindade, J., & Castro, B. (2007). Rethinking Timorese identity as a peacebuilding strategy: The Lorosa'e-Loromonu conflict from a traditional perspective. Deutsche Gesellschaft Fuer Technische Zusammenarbeit (GTZ).

United Nations. (2006). *Report of the United Nations Independent Special Commission of Inquiry for Timor-Leste*. United Nations. https://www.un.org

Wallis, J. (2013a). *Constitution-making in Timor-Leste: The role of national liberation combatants*. Routledge.

Wallis, J. (2013b). Victors, villains and victims: Capitalizing on memory in Timor-Leste. *Ethnopolitics, 12*(2), 133–160. https://doi.org/10.1080/17449057.2011.632958

Wildon, B. V. E. (2020). *Smoke and mirrors: The development of the East Timorese police 1999–2009* [Doctoral Thesis]. Canberra: The Australian National University.

Wilson, B. (2010). *Timor-Leste: Challenges of post-independence state-building and security sector reform*. Routledge.

Worldometer. (2020). Timor-Leste population. https://www.worldometers.info/world-population/timor-leste-population

9

THE GENDERED IMPACT OF CRISES

Operationalising Sri Lanka's Women, Peace and Security Agenda for Recovery and Regeneration

Lihini Ratwatte

9.1 Introduction

The year 2020 marked the 20th anniversary of the UN Security Council Resolution 1325 on Women, Peace and Security (UNSCR 1325). Although this was intended to be a milestone for women's rights and gender equality, the limited gains made in the women, peace and security agenda are at a risk of being impeded. From economic insecurity to adverse effects on health and well-being, from limited safety and security to minimal social protection, the consequences of a global crisis such as COVID-19 are heightened for women and girls – simply by virtue of their gender. In Sri Lanka, women have been at the frontlines of COVID-19 as essential workers and as healthcare providers, yet their voices in key decision-making roles have been minimal. This is observed in the low percentage of women represented in COVID-19 response teams appointed at varying stages of the pandemic in Sri Lanka (Care International, 2020).

In this chapter, I highlight that women's equal participation and leadership is vital towards an inclusive post-pandemic recovery in Sri Lanka. It is emphasised through evidence-based research that crises and conflicts have profound impacts on women and girls, often amplifying pre-existing gender inequalities. During times of conflict women and girls may experience a lack of security, loss of livelihoods, vulnerability to gender-based violence, and an increased burden of unpaid care work (UN Women, 2020f). A crisis like COVID-19 can threaten to heighten such vulnerabilities, whilst reversing gains made in securing women's rights. This is further explored through the concept of "depletion through social reproduction" – as proposed by Rai et al. (2014) – which investigates the "double burden" on women from diverse socio-economic contexts, especially during times of crisis. In this light, the chapter proposes that if Sri Lanka is to

DOI: 10.4324/9781003569084-10

leverage its women, peace and security agenda for effective COVID-19 recovery, the country must consider the contributions of women through an intersectional lens. This approach to recovery and regeneration from a crisis as proposed by Rai et al. (2019, p. 571) calls for a "moment of openness and reform," where governments, development partners, policymakers, and other key stakeholders can make a case for gender-inclusive policies that promote holistic social infrastructure, participatory policymaking, and strong accountability mechanisms to rebuild from COVID-19.

With the pandemic mimicking conflict-like dynamics and exacerbating existing inequalities, the chapter identifies how Sri Lanka's National Action Plan on Women Peace and Security (WPS NAP) can be operationalised within a post COVID-19 climate. Whilst analysing the thematic areas and strategic solutions provided in Sri Lanka's five-year WPS NAP, the chapter will propose key recommendations for policymakers and make a strong case for the implementation of the WPS NAP. The chapter determines that women must play an essential role as leaders promoting peace and security, including in accelerating socio-economic recovery and regeneration from the pandemic. It is further acknowledged that societies and economies will achieve peace and sustainable development if women can lead and participate and are guaranteed equal rights. More than 20 years since UNSCR 1325, it is vital for countries like Sri Lanka to apply the lens of women, peace and security to its COVID-19 response so that women's rights and women's leadership can be at the forefront of recovery and regeneration (Ratwatte, 2021a).

9.2   The Women, Peace and Security Agenda: Unpacking Unscr 1325

The United Nations Security Council adopted resolution 1325 on Women, Peace and Security (S/RES/1325) on 31 October 2000 to ensure that all efforts towards peacebuilding and post-conflict reconstruction are aligned with achieving gender equality. The resolution seeks to include women at all levels of decision-making and at every stage of a conflict timeline, while underpinning the needs and concerns of women in post-conflict relief and recovery. The resolution reaffirms the important role of women in the prevention and resolution of conflicts, peace negotiations, peacebuilding, peacekeeping, humanitarian response, and post-conflict reconstruction. It highlights the importance of women's equal participation and full involvement in all efforts for the maintenance and promotion of peace and security (United Nations Special Advisor on Gender Issues and Advancement of Women, 2000).

The UN Security Council Resolution 1325 (UNSCR 1325) urges actors to increase the participation of women and incorporate gender perspectives in all peace and security efforts. It also calls on all parties in conflict to take special measures to protect women and girls from gender-based violence, particularly rape and other forms of sexual abuse in situations of armed conflict. The resolution provides a number of important operational mandates, with implications for member states and the entities of the United Nations system (United Nations, 2000).

As of 31 October 2020, 20 years since the inception of UNSCR 1325, 88 countries had developed or were in the process of developing National Action Plans (NAPs) on Women, Peace and Security (WPS). Overall, 55 local action plans on WPS have been adopted in over 16 countries, although only 20 NAPs have included a budget for operationalisation at the time of adoption (UN Women, 2021a). In the case of Sri Lanka, following the completion of nation-wide consultations, the NAP on WPS received cabinet approval for implementation in February 2023 for the period of 2023–2027. The NAP was ceremoniously launched on 8 March 2023, on International Women's Day (United Nations, 2023).

However, having emerged from a 26-year armed ethnic conflict, Sri Lanka did not effectively initiate post-conflict reconciliation and regeneration through a sustainable women, peace and security agenda. From 2009 onwards, following the end of the conflict, the (then) Sri Lankan government formulated a number of instruments aimed at addressing human rights violations – including but not limited to – the Lessons Learnt and Reconciliation Commission (LLRC), the Paranagama Commission, and the Presidential Commission to Investigate into Complaints Regarding Missing Persons. In addition, multiple state institutions and policy frameworks were established to address the question on delayed reconciliation. For instance, the Office for National Unity and Reconciliation (ONUR) and the Office for Missing Persons (OMP) were established in 2016 under an overarching National Policy on Reconciliation. Subsequently, ministerial portfolios on National Integration and Reconciliation, National Coexistence Dialogue, and National Languages were established (Wakkumbura & Wijegoonawardana, 2017). Albeit having limited functions at present, the ONUR, the OMP and a separate of Office of Reparations were annexed to the National Ministry of Justice from 2019 onwards.

Despite milestones achieved at varying stages during the aftermath of the conflict in Sri Lanka, the majority of the aforementioned instruments and mechanisms were established in adherence to subsequent resolutions issued by the United Nations Office for the High Commissioner of Human Rights (UN OHCHR). There was no organic effort to effectively facilitate a holistic peace process, and at the same time, the country made limited progress with regard to transitional justice, healing and memorialisation. The exclusion of women's active contributions to Sri Lanka's post-conflict transition process is evident with the continued appraisal of exclusionary men-led mechanisms. It is within this context that a holistic "Women, Peace and Security Agenda" is vital to engage half of the country's population in key decision-making roles that will contribute to sustained peace and reconciliation.

The crisis brought on by the pandemic has offered yet another opportunity for Sri Lanka to pause and reflect on the need for women's engagement in leadership and peacebuilding aimed at recovery and regeneration, through the operationalisation of its National Action Plan on Women Peace and Security.

9.3 COVID-19 as a Crisis Mimicking Conflict-Like Dynamics

In countries across Asia and the Pacific, including in Sri Lanka, governments continued to respond to the pandemic through actions that could have negative implications for peace and security and the rights of women and girls. UN Women's research indicates that the enactment of national emergency powers, the introduction of military checkpoints, lockdowns, closed borders, and restrictions on citizens' movement and speech, all mirror a governance context similar to that of a conflict setting (UN Women, 2020f). Across the region, warlike terminology – i.e., "battling an invisible enemy" – was used to describe efforts to contain the spread of COVID-19, thus mimicking conflict-like social dynamics (UN Women, 2020f, p. 1).

In Sri Lanka, not only was the military (i.e., tri-forces) engaged in providing logistical and operational assistance, including the administration of vaccines, it also helped strategise and lead the government's coordinated COVID-19 response. The Sri Lankan Government's response to COVID-19 was headed by two entities, namely the 22-member National Operation Centre for the Prevention of the COVID-19 Outbreak (NOCPCO), and a 40-member Presidential Task Force to direct and coordinate pandemic response efforts. In March 2020, the government set up the NOCPCO to prevent the spread of the disease, with the commander of the Sri Lankan armed forces being appointed in charge of the Centre. After almost two years in operation, and with the armed forces undertaking key COVID-19 response efforts, the NOCPCO announced that it would cease functions by the end of 2021 (Sri Lanka Army, 2021). The Presidential Taskforce, which is still in effect, was established with the objective to "direct, coordinate and monitor the delivery of continuous services for the sustenance of overall community life, including the supply and distribution of food provisions in rural areas." (Government of Sri Lanka, 2020, pp. 1).

It must be noted that the above entities are largely represented by men. While NOCPCO was heavily represented by military personnel, nine out of the forty members within the Presidential Taskforce also constitute existing or retired members from security forces. Further, only four out of forty members within the Presidential Taskforce are women, with minimal to zero representation from ethnic minorities hailing from Tamil, Muslim, and Christian backgrounds. This highlights how the battle against COVID-19 is viewed not merely as a health crisis but as a conflict to be dealt with through military intervention, in which the role of health professionals is to merely "assist" the security forces. It also feeds into the rhetoric that pandemics, diseases, and natural disasters pose a grave threat to national security. It is discussed amongst security circles that a pandemic such as COVID-19 can be classified as a non-traditional threat to national security. This is witnessed in the asymmetric nature through which COVID-19 unleashes havoc across nations, while also exposing weaknesses in states' capabilities to protect their citizens (Angbo, 2021). This line of thinking aligns with the argument that the nature, scope, novelty, and complexity of COVID-19 demands an integrated national security strategy for an effective application of instruments of national power (Angbo, 2021). Within this climate, there is a natural push by governments to respond to COVID-19 by producing parallel structures made up largely of military personnel, instead of strengthening existing capacities and resources (Peiris, 2021), and engaging women and other marginalised communities.

This status quo was observed not only in Sri Lanka but across the region, with emergency powers and militarised responses being used to mitigate the pandemic. For instance, reports of police brutality emerged from some parts of India, while in Pakistan, the military was deployed to assist with pandemic preventive measures (The Nation, 2020). In Bangladesh, Prime Minister Hasina called the campaign against COVID-19 a "war" as her government reached out to the armed forces to assist nationwide efforts to "combat" the pandemic (Devnath, 2020).

However, it is important that the heavy focus on national security does not overshadow social cohesion and peace that may wither as a consequence of a crisis situation. Often, the rights of marginalised communities, including those of women, are overlooked during times of crisis and this is observed in the low representation of women and minorities in Sri Lanka's pandemic response task forces and policy priorities. This further underlines the urgency for women's engagement in leadership and peacebuilding.

9.4   The Gendered Impact of COVID-19 Through an Intersectional Lens

Crises and conflicts have profound impacts on women and girls, often amplifying pre-existing inequalities. During times of conflict, women and girls may experience a lack of security, loss of livelihoods, vulnerability to gender-based violence, and an increased burden of unpaid care work. Given the pandemic's propensity to fuel conflict-like dynamics, it can threaten to exacerbate such vulnerabilities, whilst reversing gains in women's rights (UN Women, 2020e/f).

Therefore, the impacts of crises and conflicts are never gender neutral, and COVID-19 is no exception, as women and girls are affected by the resulting socio economic fallout of the pandemic on a global scale. For instance, women make up 39% of global employment but account for 54% of overall job losses (Madgavkar et al., 2020, para 1). One reason for this greater impact on women is due to the virus significantly increasing the burden of unpaid care, which is disproportionately carried by women. In addition, women are losing their livelihoods faster as they are mostly exposed to hard-hit economic sectors such as care work and other informal employment avenues. According to an analysis commissioned by UN Women,

435 million women and girls lived on less than $1.90 a day, including 47 million being pushed into poverty as a result of COVID-19 (UN Women, 2021a).

Parallel to the economic impact, the pandemic has stifled the rights of women and girls across the board, with security-driven and emergency-centred pandemic responses shifting the focus away from fundamental rights and obligations (UN Women, 2020e/f). For instance, reports of violence against women have increased around the world, as widespread stay-at-home orders forced women to shelter in the same space as their abusers. The increasing incidents of domestic and intimate partner violence propagated during prolonged lockdowns has been dubbed a "shadow pandemic," as it coincided in many countries with a reduction in services to support victims and survivors. This is partly due to operational challenges and reduced funding for law enforcement agencies and local women's organisations, which play an essential role in service provision aimed at reducing violence against women and girls (UN Women, 2021b, paras 2, 3).

The pandemic also had a significant gendered impact in Sri Lanka. While women represent only 36% of the total labour force in Sri Lanka, 64% of employed women are engaged in the informal sector (Madurawala, 2020b, para 1). As women in the informal sector earn less and have limited access to social protection mechanisms, they were the first to lose their livelihoods when lockdowns were imposed. Sri Lankan domestic workers employed overseas – mostly women – were also stranded, with no way to return home, whilst the majority lost their jobs in their respective host countries (Weeraratne, 2020).

A study conducted by the International Finance Corporation (2020) on Sri Lanka further reported that women-led and women-run small and medium enterprises saw a decrease in sales due to the existing digital gender gap, which hindered their ability to digitise their businesses during lockdowns. Moreover, with women heading one in four households (1.4 million households) in Sri Lanka (Department of Census and Statistics, 2016), women heads of households faced a double burden with an increase in unpaid care work to support children and elderly dependents while earning an income to provide for their families (Ratwatte, 2021b, para 2).

The prolonged lockdowns have also impacted women and girls in private spaces, with emerging testimonial data on domestic and intimate partner violence (Ratnayake & Mutucumarana, 2021). Although there is currently a dearth of published data on reported cases of domestic violence during the pandemic in Sri Lanka, for many countries, records from helplines, police, and other referral service providers indicate an increase in reported cases, child maltreatment, and intimate partner violence against women – with many women being unable to access adequate support services (The Asia Foundation, 2021). However, these numbers underrepresent the scale of the problem, as data on family violence during the COVID-19 pandemic is scarce due to the lack of reporting and the inability of women to reach out for help. Undoubtedly, this is also the case for Sri Lanka where, even prior to the pandemic, a Women's Well-being Survey (2019) reported that one in five ever-partnered women in Sri Lanka had experienced physical and/ or sexual violence by an intimate partner in their lifetime.

It is evident therefore, that a crisis like COVID-19 can threaten to exacerbate existing inequalities and vulnerabilities, whilst reversing significant achievements in women's rights by decades. Against this backdrop, women's equal participation and leadership is vital towards an inclusive post-pandemic recovery in Sri Lanka.

9.5 Identifying Threats to Equality, Peace, and Social Cohesion

In addition to propagating gender inequalities, emergency environments can also amplify social tensions framed by an "us-versus-them" mentality amongst communities, thus threatening peace and social cohesion.

Sri Lanka experienced flares of ethnic and religious tensions, especially after the Easter Sunday terrorist attacks of April 2019, which killed 277 people and injured another 592. The attacks triggered a state of emergency along with the extraordinary deployment of the military (UNHCR, 2021). In the immediate aftermath of the attacks, the country's Muslim minority experienced violence and harassment followed by a government imposed a ban on *burkas* and *niqabs* (garments worn by Muslim women that cover the face and body), which increased their social marginalisation. The ban was later withdrawn, although the Human Rights Commission of Sri Lanka documented numerous cases of Muslim women wearing *burkas, niqabs,* and *hijabs* (head coverings that do not cover the face) being abused in public and denied access to public buildings such as schools, hospitals, and universities (Ganguly, 2021, paras 1, 2).

Similar patterns of violence were visible in attacks against Muslims in March 2018 (in the towns of Digana/Teldeniya and Ampara), in November 2017 (in the town of Gintota), and in 2014 (in the town of Aluthgama). Widespread perceptions suggest that such violence targeting Muslims is a post-war phenomenon since the end of the armed ethnic conflict in 2009. However, violence against Muslims dates back to the colonial era of the early 20th century in Sri Lanka (known then as Ceylon). The anti-Muslim riots of 1915 marked the deadliest violence targeting the Muslim community to date, spanning five provinces, and resulting in at least 25 deaths, four cases of sexual violence, and attacks on over 4,000 Muslim properties (Wettimuny, 2019, para 3).

Given this history and intermittent patterns of violence against minorities, Sri Lanka was immediately susceptible to hate speech, fake news, discrimination, and stigma, with minority groups and communities from low-income backgrounds being accused of being "super spreaders" or of deliberately spreading the virus (Suleiman, 2020). An incident that caught global headlines was when the Sri Lankan government moved to amend the Ministry of Health's guidelines by ordering cremations for any individual who died or was suspected to have died of COVID-19 (Amnesty International, 2020). Despite the World Health Organization

(WHO) guidance that allowed for either burials or cremations, forced cremations took place for almost a year in Sri Lanka. This guideline directly affected the final burial rites of the Muslim community, whose right to freedom of religion and belief were violated in the process. The UN special procedures condemned the move as a decision "based on discrimination, aggressive nationalism and ethnocentrism amounting to persecution of Muslims and other minorities in the country" (OHCHR, 2021). Following continued public outcry, on 5 March 2021, the government resumed burials for those deceased from COVID-19.

The spread of COVID-19 created scapegoats in communities across South Asia. For instance, in India, a group of Orthodox Muslims known as the *Tablighi Jamaat* broke quarantine curfew by organising a large gathering, which led to hundreds of positive COVID-19 cases. This incident sparked communal attacks on Muslims who had no association with the *Jammat*, and aggravated tensions in a country already grappling with the Hindu–Muslim divide as a result of far-right politics (Silva, 2020).

From an intersectional perspective therefore, the gendered impact of COVID-19 is detrimental to marginalised communities and groups. Women with diverse intersectional characteristics including, but not limited to, women from minorities, women from low-income backgrounds, women with disabilities, elderly women, girl children, transgender women, and women heads of households may face divergent and unique circumstances as a result of their lived experiences and other socio-economic factors.

9.6   Explaining "Depletion Through Social Reproduction"

The gendered impact of crises such as COVID-19 can lead to a double burden that affects women in varying degrees when observed through an intersectional lens. For instance, the economic fallout of the pandemic has exposed the lived experiences of women-headed households (WHHs). Over 25% of households in Sri Lanka (one in every four) are headed by a woman (Department of Census and Statistics, 2016). The majority of WHHs lost a spouse or a partner as a direct consequence of Sri Lanka's 26-year armed ethnic conflict that ended in 2009. WHHs were considered vulnerable even before the pandemic, as the majority of these women were only able to engage in low-paying informal employment or daily income-generation activities after the conflict. Research from UN Women (2021c) indicates that given that the majority of WHHs are engaged in informal employment, they are not entitled to employment benefits. Since they lack access to adequate social protection mechanisms, they are burdened with unpaid care and domestic work, and as a result, lose their livelihoods faster during times of crisis. Moreover, the mobility restrictions imposed due to COVID-19 severely impacted the socioeconomic security of WHHs as they faced a double burden of trying to find work while taking care of dependents at home.

A number of state and non-state actors have implemented programmes that target some of these women; however, to date there has been no inclusive national socio economic strategy focused on WHHs to be operationalised during emergency situations like COVID-19. The drafting of a National Action Plan on Women-Headed Households (WHH NAP) spearheaded by the (then) Ministry of Women and Child Affairs in 2017 is still to be finalised due to intermittent administrative and portfolio-related changes within the government.

Due to the WHH NAP still being at a draft stage, there is no nationally accepted definition for WHHs, thus prompting a plethora of de facto definitions and categorisations. The lack of a consistent definition has led to the generalisation of WHHs as a homogenous group and excluded certain vulnerable categories of WHHs, such as women with disabilities, women with spouses who are living with disabilities, divorced women, elderly women, ex-combatants, and widows of former combatants. These groups of women are loosely categorised as "war widows," and they often fall through the cracks of government welfare and social protection schemes such as *Samurdhi* (Ratwatte, 2021a). For example, following COVID-19 lockdowns and mobility restrictions, the government initiated a relief programme for ten categories of eligible beneficiaries from low-income backgrounds. However, WHHs were not considered a priority group for government concessions granted under the emergency situation resulting from the pandemic (Office of the President of Sri Lanka, 2020). The lack of a proper definition has also resulted in the absence of disaggregated data on WHHs, which makes it difficult for practitioners to identify the most vulnerable women. The latest household income and expenditure survey of 2016 categorises WHHs only by sector, province, and district (Department of Census and Statistics, 2016).

Another problematic area is the geographic focus of WHHs. Since conflict-affected areas are mainly concentrated in the north and east of the country, most research, advocacy, and media attention is concentrated on a few regions. However, WHHs are prevalent across the country, the majority being "military widows" or the living spouses of government military personnel who died during the conflict. For example, while the district of Batticaloa in the east constitutes the highest percentage of WHHs, at 32.3%, the district of Kandy in the Central Province is home to the second highest percentage of WHHs, at 31.2%. Other districts in the Southern (Galle), North Central (Anuradhapura), and North Western (Kurunegala) provinces also have high percentages of WHHs, at 28.5%, 27.2%, and 26.7%, respectively (Department of Census and Statistics, 2016). The perception is that WHHs who are military widows are economically stable, as they are eligible for a government-mandated salary and the pension of their deceased spouse, while other war widows do not receive any form of redress. Due to this prevailing notion, most targeted COVID-19 relief efforts for WHHs were heavily focused on Sri Lanka's Northern Province (UN Women, 2021c). However, research shows that in addition to significant economic burdens, including indebtedness through microfinance loans, military widows have to live under the scrutiny societal stigmas associated with widowhood and are subject to sexual bribery and other forms of sexual exploitation (Centre for Equality and Justice, 2018).

It is also pertinent to note that most "war widows" are Tamil, while the majority of "military widows" are Sinhalese. Therefore, these women fall on either side of the ethnic divide that was catalytic to the prolonged conflict. Policy practitioners often overlook the fact that by bringing these women to the forefront of policy attention, it would not only support sustainable economic development but also strengthen key peacebuilding conversations that are crucial to Sri Lanka's recovery and regeneration within the context of the pandemic (Ratwatte, 2021b, para 10).

Due to traditional gender roles and patriarchal societal values, women are often the key bearers of social reproduction in any society. Within this context, social reproduction refers to the labour that goes into reproducing, sustaining, and maintaining social life. This includes biological reproduction, unpaid care work in the household, voluntary work in the community, and emotional support for families (Hoskyns & Rai, 2007; Rai et al., 2014). Akin to the experience of WHHs, the double burden of unpaid care work, coupled with daily income-generation activities undertaken by women from unique and varying circumstances was heightened during the pandemic, while placing increased responsibilities on their shoulders at home and in other essential sectors. This has led to a depletion of women's lives, as they are labouring overtime to meet a double burden. According to findings from Rai et al. (2014) the added pressures, heightened inequalities, and double burdens faced by women during crises leads to a "depletion through social reproduction." COVID-19 has paved way for women's lives to be depleted through the pressures of social reproduction, and the lack of representation of women in key decision-making roles in Sri Lanka's pandemic response, is a further impediment.

9.7   Building a Case for Women Decision Makers

In Sri Lanka, women have been at the forefront of COVID-19 as essential frontline workers and healthcare providers, but as witnessed in the minimal representation of women in Sri Lanka's COVID-19 response taskforces, their voices in key decision-making roles remain largely absent. Research indicates that due to the invisibility of women's social reproductive labour, they are excluded from decision-making forums. Rai et al. (2014) indicate that the lack of recognition of social reproductive work harms women's entitlements. Women are treated more as recipients of welfare and a burden on the state rather than as a productive population that can lead and contribute to development.

As of 2022, Sri Lanka was ranked 110 in the Global Gender Equality index tabulated by the World Economic Forum. Countries are usually ranked against their performance in economic participation and opportunity, educational attainment, health and survival, and political empowerment. While Sri Lanka outshines its South Asian peers, particularly in women's education and health, the country is lagging behind in women's economic participation and women's political empowerment, hence resulting in a low ranking.

Although women account for 52% of the population, Sri Lanka's female labour force participation (FLFP) rate has stagnated between 30–36% for the past two decades. Moreover, 64% of employed women are engaged in the informal sector (Madurawala, 2020a, para 1). Research by the International Labour Organisation further indicates that women's work is segregated in the sectors of health and education, as most teachers, nurses, and other medical staff are female (ILO, 2016). This gender segregation is not unique to Sri Lanka, as a study in India found that women are more likely to join traditional stereotyped jobs such as teaching, nursing, and caregiving, which are socially perceived as suitable for women (Chakraborty, 2020).

It is also interesting to note that Sri Lankan women's educational attainment levels are higher when compared to men, whereby as of 2019, women undergraduates constituted 64% across all universities in Sri Lanka. Yet again, there is a visible gender segregation in certain subject domains, with more women pursuing arts (83%), management (67%), and medicine (62%), but only 23% and 45% pursuing engineering and computer science respectively (University Grants Commission, 2019). This could be an explanation as to why more women are entering universities but fewer women are retained within the labour force. The mismatch of skills for employability is witnessed due to socio cultural perceptions that discourage women from science, technology, engineering, and mathematics (STEM) subjects. Research also shows that women exit the workforce after marriage due to societal gender roles that place the responsibilities of managing the household on women's shoulders. This is further compounded by the lack of social support mechanisms such as childcare and flexible working arrangements, especially within the context of COVID-19 (International Labour Organisation, 2020).

Women's representation in decision making across senior management positions and boards of directors in listed companies has also seen a marginal increase over the years, and as of 2019, only 8.5% of listed company board directors were women – a marginal increase from that of 8.14% in 2018 (International Finance Corporation, 2019). Women's representation in Sri Lanka's national parliament has never exceeded 5.5%, and as of 2021 it was only 5.3% in a 225-member parliament (Parliament of Sri Lanka, 2021). Women were also sparsely represented in leadership positions that oversaw and facilitated Sri Lanka's post-conflict transition process. As a result, Sri Lanka is placed 181 out of 193 countries (as of 2021) by the Inter-Parliamentary Union's ranking of women's representation in parliament.

The pandemic has widened existing gaps in women's leadership that stem from deep-rooted gender inequalities. It was witnessed in Sri Lanka that many key decisions on governance, safety, and security in response to the pandemic were taken by taskforces largely represented by men. Research pertaining to pandemic leadership by two New Zealand-based scholars – Severi Luoto and Marco Varella – shows that men-led leadership approaches fail to engage the experiences and expertise of women and minority groups in decision making. Women's voices are important as they face unique challenges during a crisis or a conflict, and this allows them to provide an alternative voice based on their lived experiences. Similarly, since a crisis such as COVID-19 can become a driver of conflict, it is important that communities support women's leadership to promote peacebuilding and social cohesion. Therefore, a holistic women, peace and security agenda is vital to engage women in key decision-making roles that will contribute to sustained peace and reconciliation.

9.8 Highlighting the Need for Inclusive Policies and a Rights-Based Recovery from COVID-19

It is evident that the gendered impact of COVID-19 has highlighted the changing nature of peace and security and the increasing inequalities faced by women. Such heightened inequalities have led to a depletion of women's lives as they engage in a double burden of social reproduction. This has hindered women's meaningful participation in leadership roles, their economic empowerment, and even their safety in their own homes.

One solution is to introduce holistic regenerative policies and practices to identify women's meaningful inclusion and participation. COVID-19 exposed vulnerabilities in social, political, and economic systems, and has propelled a shift in priorities and funding across public and private sectors, with far-reaching effects on the well-being of women and girls. It is important that effective measures are undertaken to prevent the backsliding of significant gains in women's rights. Women must be included as architects as well as beneficiaries of efforts to build back stronger and better in response to the highly visible fault lines resulting from the pandemic.

Research shows that in countries with women at the helm, confirmed deaths from COVID-19 are six times lower, partly due to these leaders' faster response to the pandemic and their greater emphasis on social and environmental well-being over time (UN Women, 2020a/b). It is important therefore, that socio-economic policies and programmes are designed to be inclusive and transformative, particularly in addressing women's leadership and labour, both outside and within the home. Placing women and girls at the centre of preparedness, response, and recovery could bring about "genuine change" globally advocated by women's rights groups (UN Women, 2020d).

It is therefore pertinent that Sri Lanka's response to the pandemic be streamlined through a holistic women, peace and security agenda aimed at recovery and regeneration.

9.9 Operationalising Sri Lanka's WPS Agenda for COVID-19 Recovery and Regeneration

Through extensive island-wide consultations with women and women-led stakeholders, Sri Lanka's first ever WPS NAP proposes six thematic areas for the engagement and empowerment women in leadership and peacebuilding over a span of five years.

Thematic Priority 01: Legal, policy, and institutional reforms.

Thematic Priority 02: Addressing the impact of displacement experienced by women.

Thematic Priority 03: Addressing concerns of military widows, women ex-combatants, and female-headed households.

Thematic Priority 04: Women's protection and security.

Thematic Priority 05: Economic empowerment of women.

Thematic Priority 06: Promoting women's participation in peacebuilding, conflict prevention, conflict resolution, and in decision-making, and politics. (WPS-NAP: 2023–2027, March 2023).

The document discusses in detail the pertinent issues that infringe on the rights of women and girls and impede their active participation in peacebuilding, community cohesion, and decision-making. The implementation of the NAP can bring to light how the gendered impact of crises has highlighted the changing nature of peace and security through increasing inequalities faced by women – especially women heads of households. Often defined as a community directly impacted by Sri Lanka's armed ethnic conflict, WHHs fall through the cracks of formal development processes. Given their shared history, WHHs are considered a homogenous group, despite experiencing discrimination across varying intersectional characteristics. Therefore, the national adoption of the WPS NAP will provide an all-encompassing definition for WHHs, while recognising their unique circumstances across many intersecting factors.

The NAP can also look at ensuring ensure women's security and protection by addressing existing personal and territorial laws that are discriminatory towards women. Discriminatory laws pertaining to single women, divorced women, and their inheritance (including limitations on property rights) continue to hinder women's access to land and property, which in turn is directly linked to their economic empowerment and agency. The economic fallout of COVID-19 has made it necessary to introduce regulations on micro-finance and micro-credit companies that have led women entrepreneurs to encounter indebtedness and an inability to establish sustainable livelihoods (Gunawardana & De Silva, 2020, para 5). This is closely tied to the need for comprehensive social protection schemes for vulnerable women including WHHs.

With heightened incidence of domestic and intimate partner violence due to prolonged lockdowns, it is equally important to develop standard operating procedures to expedite court processes in a gender-responsive manner using a survivor-centred approach. Sri Lanka is also lagging behind in the implementation of particular laws for online harassment and abuse against women and girls, which has become rampant within the online infrastructure created by school-from-home and work-from-home modalities. Finally, as a country placed 181 out of 193 countries (as of 2021) by the Inter-Parliamentary Union's ranking of women's representation in parliament, it is paramount that women's leadership is cultivated through a multi-pronged approach, including capacity development, introduction of mandatory quotas, advocacy and awareness, and the engagement of men as allies of women in leadership (Ratwatte, 2021a).

It is proposed therefore, that in order to avoid the depletion of women's lives through social reproduction after a crisis like COVID-19, it is paramount that governments introduce regenerative, and gender equitable policies led by the "regenerative state." The author recommends that the Women, Peace and Security agenda can be used as a vehicle to achieve this vision.

9.10 Unpacking the "Regenerative State"

The concept of the "regenerative state," was first proposed by Shirin Rai, Jacqui True, and Maria Tanyag – a team of researchers from the University of Warwick, Monash University, and the Australian National University. The regenerative state can be used to "establish, review, or revise" policies that can address inequalities, reduce depletion, and contribute to sustainable and inclusive peace (Rai et al., 2019).

The regenerative state is an opportunity for openness and reform after a crisis or a conflict, where state and non-state actors, civil society groups, and social movements can hold the state accountable to reverse depletion and improve the quality of social reproduction. COVID-19 is such a crisis where governments, stakeholders, and policymakers can make a case for gender-inclusive policies that promote holistic development and post-pandemic recovery. Rai et al. (2019) propose that the "regenerative state can be achieved through a three-pronged approach of: 'Inclusive Social Infrastructure', 'Participatory Policymaking' and 'Strengthened Accountability Mechanisms.'"

The six thematic areas in Sri Lanka's WPS NAP can be delivered through the regenerative state as follows:

1 **Inclusive social infrastructure**

- Ensuring women's protection and security.
- Economic empowerment of women.
- Addressing the impact of displacement experienced by women.
- Addressing concerns of military widows, women ex-combatants and female-headed households.

2 **Participatory policymaking**

- Promoting women's participation in peacebuilding, conflict prevention, conflict resolution, and in decision making, and politics.

3 **Strong accountability mechanisms**

- Delivering effective legal, policy, and institutional reforms.

It is therefore proposed that Sri Lanka's WPS NAP can be operationalised to achieve this three-pronged regenerative state to build back better from COVID-19.

9.11 Concluding Remarks and Recommendations for Policymakers

Sri Lanka's efforts to formalise a five-year National Action Plan on Women Peace and Security encourage women's meaningful engagement when responding to past, present, and future crises. Whilst this chapter makes a case for the operationalisation of Sri Lanka's WPS NAP for COVID-19 recovery and regeneration, it is equally important that policymakers continue to engage with the process through accountable and transparent mechanisms. To this end, it is vital that the government implement the five-year WPS NAP utilising collaborative and intersectional strategies not only in response to COVID-19 but also in preparation for impending crises. This chapter recommends all key stakeholders to identify the WPS NAP as a national priority and as a key requirement for development and regeneration to build back stronger and better from COVID-19, and other converging crises.

With COVID-19 shedding a spotlight on the adversities faced by women and girls, it has reached a point where immediate policy attention is essential. The scope and scale of existing social protection programmes in Sri Lanka are still limited, with many poverty-targeted schemes failing to reach the most vulnerable communities. Delivering effective long-term social protection to all people – especially those that are left behind – will support communities more effectively in the aftermath of the pandemic (Ratwatte, 2021b). Furthermore, applying an intersectional and a gender-responsive lens when designing social assistance programmes and investing in women's economic empowerment is an opportunity for Sri Lanka to bounce back from a crisis.

In response to COVID-19 recovery, UN Secretary General Antonio Guterres said,

Humanity faces a stark and urgent choice: breakdown or breakthrough.

The time is *now* for a breakthrough. It has been over 20 years since the inception of UNSCR 1325, and it is essential now more than ever for countries like Sri Lanka to apply the lens of women, peace and security to the COVID-19 response so that women's rights and women's leadership can be at the forefront of development and recovery (Ratwatte, 2021a). When women lead, participate, and benefit equally in all aspects of life, societies and economies will thrive and contribute to sustainable development and peace (UN Women, 2020e). Women must play an essential role as leaders promoting peace and security, including in accelerating economic growth during any stage of a conflict cycle.

9.12 Author's Note

As the chapter was submitted for publication in 2021, the author has only viewed COVID-19 as a "crisis mimicking conflict-like dynamics." In this chapter, the author has not considered Sri Lanka's political and economic crisis that ensued in 2022. The author acknowledges that the events surrounding 2022 can present a more nuanced analysis to the arguments presented in this chapter. Hence the author will continue her research on how the Women Peace and Security Agenda can respond to Sri Lanka's converging crises.

Bibliography

Amnesty International. (2020). Religious minorities must have their final rites respected. https://www.amnesty.org/en/latest/news/2020/04/sri-lanka-religious-minorities-must-have-their-final-rites-respected/

Angbo, P. K. (2021). National security redesign after the COVID–19: Nepali Army's security priority in response to the global pandemics. *Unity Journal, 2*, 163–174. https://doi.org/10.3126/unityj.v2i0.38823

Asia Foundation. (2021). Local communities and the Sri Lanka police support sensitive responses to gender-based violence during the Covid-19 pandemic. https://asiafoundation.org/2021/02/26/local-communities-and-the-sri-lanka-police-support-sensitive-responses-to-gender-based-violence-during-the-covid-19-pandemic/

Care International. (2020). Where are the women? The conspicuous absence of women in COVID-19 response teams and plans, and why we need them. https://www.care-international.org/files/files/CARE_COVID-19-womens-leadership-report_June-2020.pdf

Centre for Equality and Justice. (2018). Sexual bribery of military widows in Sri Lanka: Anuradhapura, Kurunegala and Galle Districts. https://cejsrilanka.org/wp-content/uploads/Sexual-Bribery-Of-Military-Widows-English.pdf

Center for Policy Alternatives. (2018). Human rights commitments made by the government of Sri Lanka and ways forward. https://www.cpalanka.org/wp-content/uploads/2018/02/HR-Commitments-_final-.pdf

Chakraborty, S. (2020). Gender wage differential in public and private sectors in India. *Indian Journal of Labour Economics, 63*, 765–780. https://doi.org/10.1007/s41027-020-00246-1

Daily Mirror. (2021, November 26). Validations begin for National Action Plan on women, peace and security. (Online). https://www.dailynews.lk/2021/11/26/local/265704/validations-begin-national-action-plan-women-peace-and-security

Department of Census and Statistics. (2016). Female headed households by sector, province and district. http://www.statistics.gov.lk/Resource/en/GenderStatistics/Special_Concerns/FemaleHeadedHouseholdsBySector,ProvinceAndDistrict2016.pdf

Department of Census and Statistics. (2020). Women's Wellbeing Survey – 2019: Findings from Sri Lanka's first dedicated National Survey on Violence against women and girls. http://www.statistics.gov.lk/Resource/refference/WWS_2019_Final_Report

Devnath, A. (2020, March 21). Bangladesh readies itself for the COVID-19 battle. *The Hindu.* (Online). https://www.thehindu.com/news/international/despatch-from-dhaka-bangladesh-readies-itself-for-the-covid-19-battle/article31130228.ece

Ganguly, M. (2021). Sri Lanka face covering ban latest blow for Muslim women: Discriminatory measure targets marginalized population. *Human Rights Watch.* https://www.hrw.org/node/378644/printable/print

Government of Sri Lanka. (2020, March 26). Gazette extraordinary of the democratic socialist Republic of Sri Lanka. https://policy.asiapacificenergy.org/node/4335

Gunawardana, S., & De Silva, N. (2020). Rethinking microfinance in post-war Sri Lanka: Mobilisation and call for reform. *Monash Gender Peace and Security Blog.* https://www.monash.edu/arts/gender-peace-security/news-and-events/articles/rethinking-microfinance-in-post-war-sri-lanka-mobilisation-and-call-for-reform

Guterres, A. (2021). Humanity faces a stark and urgent choice: Breakdown or breakthrough. *United Nations Sustainable Development Group – Action 2030 Blog.* https://unsdg.un.org/latest/blog/humanity-faces-stark-and-urgent-choice-breakdown-or-breakthrough

Hoskyns, C., & Rai, S. (2007). Recasting the global political economy: Counting women's unpaid work. *New Political Economy, 12*(3), 297–317. https://doi.org/10.1080/13563460701485268

Inter Parliamentary Union. (2021). *Women in politics.* https://www.ipu.org/women-in-politics-2021

International Finance Cooperation. (2019). Women on boards of companies listed on the Colombo stock exchange. Second Edition. https://www.ifc.org/wps/wcm/connect/382daf0e-82e8-40f7-9f04-6beaab5a8872/Women_on_Boards_of_Companies_Listed_on_the_Colombo_Stock_Exchange_2nd_edition.pdf?MOD=AJPERES

International Finance Cooperation. (2020). Gendered impacts of COVID-19 on small and medium-sized enterprises in Sri Lanka. https://www.ifc.org/wps/wcm/connect/region__ext_content/ifc_external_corporate_site/south+asia/resources/gendered+impacts+of+covid19+on+small+and+medium+sized+enterprises+in+sri+lanka

International Labour Organisation – Office for Sri Lanka and Maldives. (2016). Factors affecting women's labour force participation in Sri Lanka. https://www.ilo.org/wcmsp5/groups/public/—asia/—ro-bangkok/—ilo-colombo/documents/publication/wcms_551675.pdf

Jayasekara, K. M. S. D., & Naciri, M. (2021). Op-Ed: Why 'women, peace & security' for COVID-19 recovery? *UN Women Asia Pacific.* https://asiapacific.unwomen.org/en/news-and-events/stories/2021/03/op-ed-why-women-peace-and-security-for-covid-19-recovery#about

Luoto, S., & Varella, M. A. C. (2021). Pandemic leadership: Sex differences and their evolutionary developmental origins. *Frontiers in Psychology, 12,* 618. https://doi.org/10.3389/fpsyg.2021.633862

Madgavkar, A., White, O., Krishnan, M., Mahajan, D., & Azcue, X. (2020). *COVID-19 and gender equality: Countering the regressive effects.* McKinsey & Company. https://www.mckinsey.com

Madurawala, S. (2019). Greater social protection for Sri Lankan women through better jobs: Role of technology and innovation. *Talking Economics.* https://www.ips.lk/talkingeconomics/2019/03/08/3044/

Madurawala, S. (2021). Social perceptions on the role of women must change. *Talking Economics.* https://www.ips.lk/talkingeconomics/2021/03/19/social-perceptions-on-the-role-of-women-must-change/

Madurawala, S. (2020a). *Challenges and opportunities for gender equality in South Asia.* Routledge.

Madurawala, S. (2020b). *Gender equality and economic recovery in post-COVID-19 South Asia.* United Nations Development Programme. https://www.undp.org

Ministry of Women and Child Affair. (2023). National action plan on women, peace and security (Sri Lanka) 2023 – 2027. http://www.childwomenmin.gov.lk/news/post/7643

Office of the President of Sri Lanka. (2020). More concessions to public in the face of COVID-19 outbreak. https://www.president.gov.lk/more-concessions-to-public-in-the-face-of-covid-19-outbreak/

Office of the Special Adviser on Gender Issues and Advancement of Women. (2000). Land-mark resolution on women, peace and security. https://www.un.org/womenwatch/osagi/wps/

OHCHR. (2021). Sri Lanka: Compulsory cremation of COVID-19 bodies cannot con-tinue, say UN experts. https://www.ohchr.org/EN/NewsEvents/Pages/DisplayNews.aspx?NewsID=26686&LangID=E

Parliament of Sri Lanka. (2021). Lady members. https://www.parliament.lk/lady-members

Rai, S. M., Hoskyns, C., & Thomas, D. (2014). Depletion: The cost of social reproduction. *International Feminist Journal of Politics*, *16*(1), 86–105. https://doi.org/10.1080/1461 6742.2013.789641

Rai, S., True, J., & Tanyag, M. (2019). From depletion to regeneration: Addressing structural and physical violence in post-conflict economies. *Social Politics*, *26*(4), 562–585.

Ratnayake, C., & Mutucumarana, T. (2021). Adding fuel to the fire: The dramatic rise in do-mestic violence during COVID-19. *Groundviews.* https://groundviews.org/2021/09/22/adding-fuel-to-the-fire-the-dramatic-rise-in-domestic-violence-during-covid-19/

Ratwatte, L. (2021a). Spotlight on Sri Lanka's women headed households affected by COVID-19. *The Diplomat.* https://thediplomat.com/2021/06/spotlight-on-sri-lankas-women-headed-households-affected-by-covid-19/

Ratwatte, L. (2021b). What needs to change for the 5% of women in politics and the 52% population of women in Sri Lanka – 2. *Women For Politics.* https://www.womenforpoli tics.com/post/what-needs-to-change-for-the-5-of-women-in-politics-and-the-52-popula tion-of-women-in-sri-lanka-2

Silva, K. T. (2020). Identity, infection and fear: A preliminary analysis of COVID-19 drivers and responses in Sri Lanka. *International Centre for Ethnic Studies (ICES).* http://ices.lk/publications/identity-infection-and-fear/

Sri Lanka Army. (2021). NOCPCO operations formally culminate to undertake one more na-tional task. https://alt.army.lk/covid19/content/nocpco-operations-formally-culminate-undertake-one-more-national-task

Suleiman, O. (2020, May 20). Like India, Sri Lanka is using Coronavirus to Stigmatise Muslims. *Al Jazeera.* (Online). https://www.aljazeera.com/opinions/2020/5/20/like-india-sri-lanka-is-using-coronavirus-to-stigmatise-muslims

The Nation. (2020, March 29). Army troops deployed across Pakistan to contain COVID-19 outbreak. (Online). https://nation.com.pk/29-Mar-2020/army-troops-deployed-across-pakistan-to-contain-covid-19-outbreak

United Nations General Assembly. (2021). *Promoting reconciliation, accountability and Human Rights in Sri Lanka. Annual Report of the United Nations High Commissioner for Human Rights submitted at the Forty-sixth session of the Human Rights Counsil held between 22 February – 19 March 2021.* https://undocs.org/A/HRC/46/20

United Nations Security Council. Resolution 1325. (2000). https://www.un.org/womenwatch/osagi/wps/

University Grants Commission. (2019). Sri Lanka University Statistics 2019. https://ugc.ac.lk/index.php?option=com_content&view=article&id=2220%3A sri-lanka-university-statistics-2019&catid=55%3Areports&Itemid=42&lang=en

UN Women. (2020a). Addressing the economic fallout of COVID-19: Pathways and policy options for a gender-responsive recovery. https://eca.unwomen.org/en/digital-library/publications/2020/06/policy-brief-addressing-the-economic-fallout-of-covid-19

UN Women. (2020b). Covid-19 and the care economy: Immediate action and structural transformation for a gender-responsive recovery. https://www.unwomen.org/en/digital-library/publications/2020/06/policy-brief-covid-19-and-the-care-economy

UN Women. (2020c). Hidden challenges: Addressing sexual bribery in Sri Lanka. https://asiapacific.unwomen.org/en/news-and-events/stories/2020/12/hidden-challenges-addressing-sexual-bribery-in-sri-lanka

UN Women. (2020d). Standing up to the challenge: Response to the COVID-19 pandemic in Asia and the Pacific. https://asiapacific.unwomen.org/en/digital-library/publications/2021/02/standing-up-to-the-challenge-response-to-the-covid-19-pandemic-in-asia-and-the-pacific

UN Women. (2020e). UN secretary-general's policy brief: The impact of COVID-19 on women. https://www.unwomen.org/en/digital-library/publications/2020/04/policy-brief-the-impact-of-covid-19-on-women

UN Women. (2020f). Women, peace and security and Covid-19 in Asia and the Pacific. https://asiapacific.unwomen.org/en/digital-library/publications/2020/03/women-peace-and-security-and-covid-19-in-asia-pacific

UN Women. (2021a). Facts and figures: Women, peace, and security. https://www.unwomen.org/en/what-we-do/peace-and-security/facts-and-figures

UN Women. (2021b). Measuring the shadow pandemic: Violence against women during COVID-19. https://data.unwomen.org/publications/vaw-rga

UN Women. (2021c). Supporting female heads of households to overcome COVID-19's economic toll in Sri Lanka. https://www.unwomen.org/en/news/stories/2021/2/feature-women-overcoming-covid-19-economic-toll-in-sri-lanka

United Nations. (2023). Sri Lanka adopts first National Action Plan on women, peace and security. https://srilanka.un.org/en/222596-sri-lanka-adopts-first-national-action-plan-women-peace-and-security

Wakkumbura, M., & Wijegoonawardana, N. (2017). A study on reconciliation of post-war peacebuilding in Sri Lanka. *Colombo Journal of Multi-Disciplinary Research, 3*(1), 23–38. http://doi.org/10.4038/cjmr.v3i1.25

Weeraratne, B. (2020). Repatriation and replacement of lost foreign jobs: Handling labour migration in Sri Lanka during COVID-19. *Talking Economics*. https://www.ips.lk/talkingeconomics/2020/05/14/repatriation-and-replacement-of-lost-foreign-jobs-handling-labour-migration-in-sri-lanka-during-covid-19/

World Economic Forum. (2022). *Global gender gap report*. https://www3.weforum.org/docs/WEF_GGGR_2021.pdf

10

ISLAMIC SOCIAL FINANCE CONTRIBUTION IN PANDEMIC COVID-19

Evidence from Indonesia

Efri Syamsul Bahri, Hendro Wibowo, Pamungkas Hendra Kusuma, and Nur Efendi

10.1 Introduction

The COVID-19 pandemic was first reported in Wuhan, China (Yi et al., 2021). The World Health Organization (WHO, 2020a) stated that, in December 2019, there was a surge in respiratory diseases caused by the new coronavirus detected in China. On 30 January 2020 the WHO declared COVID-19 a global public health emergency. Furthermore, on 11 March, in the WHO report, the director-general of the WHO stated that COVID-19 was a pandemic. According to the WHO, as of 17 February the Indonesian government had reported 893 confirmed cases. In its latest report, WHO (2020b) mentioned that as of 17 February, the Indonesian government reported 1,243,646 (9,687 new) cases of confirmed COVID-19, including 33,788 deaths. A total of 1,047,676 cases were recovered from 510 districts across the 34 provinces.

Haleem et al. (2020) explained that COVID-19 has affected daily life and slowed global economic activity. Fitriani (2020) found that the COVID-19 pandemic has affected various aspects of life, including the economy. Fernandes (2020) revealed that global recession is inevitable. Therefore, Rizal and Mukaromah (2020) argued that poverty is a macroeconomic problem during a pandemic.

According to government data published by the BPS (2020) in Indonesia, there were 26.42 million poor people in March 2020. It shows that poverty has increased by 1.63 million people compared to poverty in September 2019 of 24.79 million people (Darmawan & Desiana, 2021). Furthermore, based on a survey performed by the Badan Pusat Statistik (BPS) (2020), 2.52 per cent of workers were laid off because their companies were affected by COVID-19, and increased to 18.34 per cent were laid off. Rizal and Mukaromah (2020) supported these findings.

DOI: 10.4324/9781003569084-11

The research results by Susilawati et al. (2020) illustrate that the COVID-19 pandemic affects the livelihood of the Indonesian economy. Susilawati et al. (2020) described several sectors affected by COVID-19, including transportation, tourism, and trade. However, the economic sector is considerably affected by COVID-19, especially the household economy. Fitriani (2020) finds that stopping economic activity results in reduction in income. Fitriani (2020) mentions that the impact of the COVID-19 pandemic is the loss of employment which affects vulnerable groups.

Mustahiq is an element of the society affected by COVID-19. According to Fitriani (2020), people are unable to meet their daily needs. This is because they lost their income. Fitriani (2020) classified Mustahiq affected by the COVID-19 pandemic into vulnerable groups, small and medium business groups, and groups with disabilities. Islamic social finance played a strategic role in overcoming the Mustahiq's burden. In Indonesia, Islamic social finance collects and distributes funds sourced from Islamic social finance, namely, zakat, infaq/alm, waqf, and humanitarian donations. Olanrewaju et al. (2020) explains that Islamic social finance, which comes from zakat, infaq/alms, and waqf, is an Islamic system that represents a robust socioeconomic structure that redistributes wealth to reduce poverty in society. In a recent article, Ascarya (2020a) concluded that Islamic social finance could be an explanation for handling COVID-19 economic consequences by using zakat, donations, and alms to meet consumptive needs and endowments used in health infrastructure assistance. This analysis is in line that of with Rizal and Mukaromah (2020), who state that zakat, infaq/alms, and waqf funds can increase purchasing power and overcome poverty.

Bailyail (2020) stated that the disbursement of zakat infaq/alms during a pandemic is a hope for people struggling economically. Research results from Ainol-Basirah and Siti-Nabiha (2020) found that the waqf project has made positive progress. It can be seen from the cash waqf initiative that it makes it possible to build comprehensive economic sustainability (Ainol-Basirah & Siti-Nabiha, 2020). Ahmed (2007) explained that waqf-based Islamic MFIs can also provide microfinance and facilitate wealth creation for the poor.

Several studies have examined the role and potential of Islamic social finances. However, research on this topic has rarely been conducted to explain the contribution of Islamic social finance to helping Mustahiq during the COVID-19 pandemic. This study describes the contribution of Islamic social finance to Indonesia during the COVID-19 pandemic.

10.2   Literature Review

10.2.1   Islamic Social Finance

According to Alam (2020), social finance models include waqf, zakat, and qard hassan. Olanrewaju et al. (2020) described the Islamic social finance (ISF) of zakat, sadaqah, and waqf as an old Islamic system. This represents a resilient socioeconomic structure that redistributes wealth in order to reduce poverty. Olanrewaju et al. (2020) argued that ISF represents various institutions under Islam's umbrella to protect social welfare and individual interests by stimulating economic activity to increase public happiness. Zain and Ali (2017) argued that Islamic social finance is social finance or social investment that follows Sharia rules and principles. Julia et al. (2020) supported these findings.

Obaidullah and Shirazi (2017) define Islamic social finance as a sector consisting of traditional Islamic institutions based on philanthropy – zakat, sadaqah, and waqf; institutions based on cooperation, for example, qard and kafalah; as well as contemporary Islamic microfinance institutions. Ascarya (2020) illustrates this in institutional forms including baitul maal, zakat, waqf, and Sharia micro finance.

According to Julia et al. (2020), Islamic social finance practices can be divided into three categories. The first group is based on the opinions of Abduh (2019) and Azman and Ali (2019), namely traditional Islamic instruments based on philanthropy, such as zakat, alms, and waqf. The second group is based on the Islamic Social Finance Report 2015 (Obaidullah & Shirazi, 2015), namely, cooperative-based foundations, such as qard al hasana and kafala. The third group comprises other modern forms of Islamic financial service. For example, Tahiri Jouti (2019) argued that Islamic microfinance, sukuk, and takaful waqf. Azman and Ali (2019) stated that this form of crowdfunding is Islamic crowdfunding, which has a social impact.

10.2.2 Zakat Principle

According to Qardawi (1973), zakat is not worshipped purely. However, zakat is also a determined right of the poor and a material component of society's social and economic systems (Qardawi, 1973). Qardawi (1973) explained that zakat, as defined in Sharia, is determined in Medina. Qardawi (1973) argues that zakat is a recognised and determined obligation, determined by the Sharia, so that Muslims can know the ratios, conditions, and exceptions of this obligation. The purpose of zakat is also well defined in the Alquran and in more detail in the Sunnah (Qardawi, 1973).

Generally, zakat is divided into two types: zakat fitrah and zakat maal. Zakat maal comprises income/professional zakat, trade zakat, stock zakat, and company zakat. Zakat management entities manage all the zakat funds. In Indonesia, according to Law No.23 of 2011, zakat management is defined as the planning, implementation, and coordination of zakat collection, distribution, and utilisation. This law states that zakat management in Indonesia is conducted by two zakat management entities: the National Amil Zakat Agency and Amil Zakat institution. Baznas are nonstructural government institutions with authority to manage zakats at the national level. The LAZ is a zakat management entity initiated by the community to assist baznas in collecting, distributing, and utilising zakat funds.

10.2.3 Wakaf Principle

According to Hidayatullah (2016), waqf refers to holding something whose benefits are good. Ahmed (2007) argues that waqf is called Sadaqah Jariyah. Pitchay et al. (2018) explain that Sharia recognises waqf as a voluntary zakat fund for social and economic development. In contrast to other types of Islamic social finance, consumable time has permanent immutability (Ahmed, 2007).

In the guide on Cash Waqf Linked Sukuk (CWLS) SERI SWR001, the Ministry of Finance (2020) explains that, according to fikih experts (Syafii and Ahmad bin Hambal), waqf means releasing waqf property from waqif ownership after the waqf procedure is perfect. Thus, a wakif may not do anything to donate assets.

Hidayatullah (2016) explained that the term "waqf" was not explicitly stated in the Alquran. Instead, scholars of fiqh make general verses based on waqf law in Islam, such as verses that discuss goodness, sadaqah, infaq, and amal jariyah (Hidayatullah, 2016). Ascarya (2020) argued that the division of waqf types in the contemporary period resulted from ijtihad from past sources. Therefore, waqf activities can be divided into several groups, based on various perspectives.

In a recent article, Ascarya (2020) explained that from a return orientation perspective, waqf can be divided into three categories: social waqf with a not-for-profit orientation, productive social combination waqf with no orientation, and productive waqf with for-profit orientation. The results were then used for social activities. From a form perspective, Pitchay et al. (2018) found that waqf could be in the form of money necessary for economic development to overcome unemployment.

According to Pitchay et al. (2018), waqf was a voluntary Islamic donation recommended by the Prophet Muhammad in the early Islamic era. According to Ahmed (2007), one use of a cash waqf is to provide microfinance to the poor. The purpose of waqf is for a wider community, including providing religious services and socioeconomic assistance to segments in need, the poor, education, the environment, science, and other needs (Ahmed, 2007). Ahmed (2007) argued that an essential feature of waqf is related to its purpose, namely, the idea of a birr (charity for good).

Yumarni and Suhartini (2019) explained that the principle of using waqf objects is the basis for the existence of the waqf itself. Yumarni and Suhartini (2019) argued that, in waqf worship, the value of a reward is sustainably received by a wakif. Although his wakif had passed away, the rewards continued to flow. Therefore, waqf objects can be categorised as having lasting benefits and the community can use waqf objects. For example, people donate land to established public schools (Yumarni & Suhartini, 2019).

A recent study by Faturohman et al. (2021) found that during the COVID-19 pandemic, waqf could increase economic activity by using waqf assets for various purposes, such as education and infrastructure. Furthermore, the research results of Thaker et al. (2020) proposed a model of integrated cash waqf micro-enterprise investment (ICWME-I) for micro-enterprises for human capital development. Therefore, it is the correct initiative to increase micro-enterprises through the HCD program by ensuring the proper utilisation of cash waqf funds to build a modern, subsidised cost training centre with state-of-the-art facilities. This is also supported by research by Nurjannah and Abdulllah (2020) that cash waqf can help establish a waqf hospital specifically for COVID-19 victims, waqf personal protective equipment, waqf masks, waqf polyclinics, waqf isolation houses, funding for vaccines, and helping microentrepreneurs sustain businesses affected by the pandemic.

10.2.4 Fatwa, the Indonesian Ulema Council

During the COVID-19 epidemic, the Indonesian Ulema Council (MUI) issued Fatwa Number 23 of 2020 concerning zakat infaq/alms assets to cope with the COVID-19 outbreak and its impact. In the Fatwa, the MUI explained five issuance issues. One point of consideration is that the impact of the COVID-19 outbreak is not only on health but also on social, economic, cultural, and other aspects of life.

In the Fatwa, MUI made four decisions. Overcoming the COVID-19 outbreak and its impacts are efforts aimed at preventing the spread of COVID-19, caring for and treating victims of COVID-19, reducing the death rate, limiting the transmission and spread of the disease so that the outbreak does not spread to other areas, and helping Muslims affected by COVID-19. Thus, the use of Islamic social finance funds in ZIS for handling COVID-19 has received approval from the MUI.

10.2.4.1 Method

This study used a qualitative descriptive method. Data were obtained from several Islamic social finance institutions in Indonesia that have played a role in handling COVID-19. Data come from Islamic social finance institutions that have played a role in delivering COVID-19 assistance in Indonesia, including The National Board of Zakat (Baznas), the Indonesian Waqf Board (BWI), LAZ Dewan Dakwah, LAZ Rumah Zakat, and Paguyuban Sakinah Berkah Mandiri. Data were obtained through documentation, literature review, and internet searches. The literature review was based on reference journal articles. The Islamic social finance research data analysis was conducted using a descriptive approach.

10.3 Results and Discussion

10.3.1 The Entity of Islamic Social Finance

In Indonesia, Islamic social finance comprises zakat management entities and waqf managers. The first was the zakat management entity. The zakat management entity functions as an amil. The Zakat management entity consists of the National Board of Zakat (Baznas), Baznas Province, Baznas Regency/City, and Amil Zakat institution (LAZ). LAZ exists in national, provincial, and district/city areas. According to the national Zakat statistics published by Baznas (2019), Indonesia has 572 zakat management entities. The results are shown in Table 10.1.

TABLE 10.1 Number of zakat management entities in Indonesia

Entity Category	Scope of Operation	Number of Units
Baznas	Nasional	1
Baznas Province	Provinsi	34
Baznas Regency/City	Kabupaten/Kota	456
LAZ National Level	Nasional	26
LAZ Province Level	Provinsi	18
LAZ Regency/City Level	Kabupaten/Kota	37

Source: Baznas (2019)

Table 10.1 shows that zakat management in Indonesia is carried out by 572 entities spread across 34 provinces and 456 districts/cities. Then, entities from government agencies, namely, Baznas, are carried out by entities from the LAZ community.

An equally good distribution should ideally follow good zakat collection. In the context of COVID-19, Zakat distribution was beneficial for reducing the detrimental impact of Mustahiq during the COVID-19 period. Therefore, the MUI Fatwa Number 23 of 2020 was the basis for the distribution of zakat Mustahiq during the COVID-19 pandemic. The fatwa explained zakat, infaq, and sadaqah in handling COVID-19 and their impact. Responding to COVID-19, zakat management entities throughout Indonesia formed the COVID-19 Crisis Centre, aiming to help prevent the spread of COVID-19, especially for Mustahiq, who are among vulnerable groups. Through this collaboration, all zakat management entities worked together to help all community members affected by the COVID-19 pandemic. This synergy is carried out through various programs, including economy, health, preaching, and education.

The second type is comprised of waqf management entities. The waqf management entity functions as the Nazhir of the waqf. The Indonesian Waqf Board is based on an independent institution's regulations for developing a waqf. According to BWI, there are currently 272 Nadzir waqf entities. Based on these rules, there are six duties and functions of BWI: 1) guiding Nazhir in managing and developing waqf assets, 2) managing and developing waqf assets on a national and international scale, 3) giving approval and/or permission for changes in the designation and status of waqf assets, 4) dismissing and replacing Nazhir, 5) approving the exchange of waqf assets, and 6) providing advice and considerations to the government in formulating policies in the area of waqf funds.

From research results, Hafizah (2020) offers seven solutions to the Islamic social, economic, and financial systems in handling the COVID-19 pandemic, as follows:

1 Distribution of direct cash assistance originating from zakat, donations, and alms.
2 Strengthening waqf includes cash waqf, productive waqf, sukuk related to waqf, and waqf related to infrastructure.

3 Providing superior business capital assistance to the business sector or micro, small, and medium-sized enterprises (MSMEs).
4 Qardhul Hasan scheme assistance.
5 Increasing Islamic economic and financial literacy; increase in Islamic economic and financial literacy.
6 Development of Islamic financial technology.
7 Giving awareness to the Muslim community that even economic activity is inseparable from obedience to Allah.

Hafizah (2020) states that Islamic social finance entities in Indonesia have many programs and activities. This is reinforced by Fatwa Number 23 of 2020, concerning the use of zakat assets. The Infaq/Alms (ZIS) COVID-19 outbreak and its impact. Thus, Islamic social finance entities can make maximum effort to collect and distribute zakat and waqf funds.

10.3.2   The Role of Islamic Social Finance

There are three categories of Islamic social finance in Indonesia: Zakat fund management entities, waqf fund management entities, and humanitarian fund management entities. In this study, five Islamic social finance entities contributed to handling COVID-19 in order to help Mustahiq. These five entities included Baznas, BWI, LAZ Dewan Dakwah, LAZ Rumah Zakat, and Paguyuban Sakinah Berkah Mandiri. However, these entities represent only thousands of Islamic social finances that contributed to Mustahiq during the COVID-19 pandemic. The roles of each Islamic social finance system are listed in Table 10.2.

Table 10.2 shows that zakat management entities have contributed to handling the COVID-19 outbreak. First, Baznas is a nonstructural government institution. The funds managed by the Baznas came from Zakat and Infaq/Alms. The collected funds were then distributed to the Mustahiq. During the COVID-19 pandemic, the Baznas contributed to the distribution of various programs in the Maqashid Sharia model. This is done to safeguard religion, reason, property, and the soul (Sariyati, 2020).

Programs to protect religion during the COVID-19 pandemic included funeral services, washing mosque carpets, and distributing prayer mats. In addition, there are programs to maintain reason in online education, strengthen radio-based communication tools, and provide public education. Programs for safeguarding assets include ready-to-eat food distribution, cash for work, family logistics packages, Mustahiq cash assistance, direct cash assistance, public kitchens, and support for rice and fruit. Life-saving programs include the following activities: spraying disinfectants, distribution of hands-on filters, distribution of masks, healthy sinks, health services, ambulance alerts, support for personal protective equipment, ventilators, and X-rays, isolation observation rooms, and hospital support.

To operate all programs during the COVID-19 period, Baznas implemented two zakat distribution strategies: a special distribution program and a security

TABLE 10.2 Profile of Islamic social finance entities

No	Entity	Description
1	The National Board of Zakat (Baznas)	The National Board of Zakat (Baznas) is formed based on the Decree of the President of the Republic of Indonesia No. 8 of 2001 as a nonstructural government institution, independent and accountable to the president through the minister of religion. Baznas is responsible for managing zakat based on Islamic law, trust, benefit, justice, legal certainty, integration, and accountability.
2	The Indonesian Waqf Board (BWI)	The Indonesian Waqf Board (BWI) is an independent state institution established under Law Number 41 of 2004 concerning Waqf. BWI aims to develop and advance waqf in Indonesia.
3	LAZ Dewan Dakwah	LAZ Dewan Dakwah is a national amil zakat institution established by the Dewan Dakwah Foundation. LAZ Dewan Dakwah carries out fundraising and distributes zakat, infaq/alms funds to support dakwah programs' implementation in scholarships for education, dakwah interior, empowerment of people, humanity, and health.
4	Rumah Zakat	Rumah Zakat is a sharia social and financial institution that focuses on philanthropy. The types of funds managed consist of zakat funds, alms, and other social funds. The funds collected are then channelled into community empowerment programs through four main groups, namely Champion Smiles (education), Senyum Sehat (health), Senyum Mandiri (economic empowerment), and Smile Lestari (environmental sustainability initiatives).
5	Paguyuban Sakinah Berkah Mandiri	Paguyuban Sakinah Berkah Mandiri consists of mothers with economic backgrounds from underprivileged families. They are around the Antapani-Arcamanik area of Bandung. The existence of this association has helped lighten the burden of these family fighters.

Source: From: Badan Zakat Nasional (BAZNAS) (2020).

program. Particular distribution programs were in the form of health emergencies with curative health services. Thus, through food security assistance, an economic emergency program increases purchasing power. A security program was implemented to increase the adaptability of the Mustahiq during the COVID-19 pandemic in the form of business models, marketing, and mentoring. Output adaptation was achieved by innovating Mustahiq's products. For example, tailors could use clothing to produce masks. There is also a form of honey production needed to maintain health during the CIVID-19 period.

The second was the Indonesian Waqf Board. During the COVID-19 pandemic, BWI launched two programs to help Muslims and the general public in Indonesia: the Waqf Peduli Indonesia (KALISA) program and the Cash Waqf Linked Sukuk

(CWLS) program. KALISA is a waqf-invested collection programme. Investments are used in social and emergency programmes to respond to COVID-19. The KALISA program comprises three categories. The first category was the KALISA donation programme for emergency ventilators. The funds collected to provide ventilators in hospitals have become a reference for treating COVID-19 patients.

The second category was KALISA's donations to continue living. The funds collected were used to assist the parents of underprivileged students in Indonesia, whose social and economic conditions were affected by COVID-19. The third category was Kalisa Peduli inland ulama. The funds raised were used to provide cash assistance to clerics in the interiors affected by the COVID-19 pandemic. Finally, the Waqf Bangun Negeri program (WAKABRI) is a collection of cash waqf with a program for distributing cash waqf investment results for infrastructure development in the health, education, and social sectors, such as the construction of hospitals, provision of educational facilities and infrastructure or other social needs of the community.

The CWLS program is a form of cash waqf investment in state Sukuk whose rewards are channelled by Nazhir (manager of funds and waqf activities) to finance social programs and provide economic empowerment of the people. The distribution of State Sharia Securities rewards social activities, including social infrastructure and waqf assets. Retail CWLS is managed based on Sharia principles; does not contain elements of usury, gharar (obscurity), or maysir (gambling); and has obtained a statement of Sharia conformity from the National Sharia Council and the Indonesian Ulama Council (Number B-578/DSN-MUI/IX/2020, 29 September 2020) (Ministry of Finance, 2020).

According to the Ministry of Finance (2020), the objectives of the CWLS include 1) facilitating the community to have safe and productive waqf money; 2) developing innovations in the field of finance and social investment in Indonesia; 3) encouraging inclusive and sustainable economic growth; 4) supporting the National Waqf Movement, helping social investment development, and developing a productive waqf in Indonesia; and 5) strengthening the cash waqf ecosystem in Indonesia (Table 10.3).

Third, the LAZ Dewan Dakwah focused on the health, food, and dakwah aspects. LAZ Dewan Dakwah is a national-level amil zakat institution confirmed by the government through the Decree of the Minister of Religion No. 712, dated 2 December 2016. LAZ Dewan Dakwah collected the zakat and infaq/alms. These funds support dakwah programs such as educational scholarships, interior dakwah, community empowerment, humanity, and health.

During the COVID-19 pandemic, Dewan Dakwah contributed to Dakwah's health. The aid was distributed across eight items: hand sanitiser, herbal COVID medicines, disinfectant spray, prayer mats, personal protective equipment, staple foods, portable sinks, and alms food. LAZ Dewan Dakwah also conducts socialisation and education for the public. One of these locations is on Bur Island. Activities were conducted in the form of 3M education (washing hands before doing

TABLE 10.3 Optimisation of CWLS to finance social projects

No	Categories	Social Project
1	Healthy Home/ Clinic	Provision of free pre-service health facilities for the poor, for example, the Ahmad Wardi Eye Hospital
2	Social Infrastructure	Financing of social infrastructure and social programs in the regions include an exploration of productive waqf in Riau Province.
3	Social activities	Development of an endowment fund for social institutions, such as the BPKH Benefit Fund
4	Corporate Social Responsibility	Development of CSR funds for social activities, for example, corporate and BUMN CSR Funds
5	Plantation/Animal Husbandry	Utilisation of non-productive land for livestock/ plantations, which has the potential of 420 thousand ha., for example. Waqf for Dompet Dhuafa Plantation
6	Health services	Free health services for the poor, for example, free cataract surgery
7	Empowerment of MSMEs	Empowerment of MSMEs, for example, productive UMKM Waqf by Waqf Houses
8	Free Umrah	Free Umrah program for Alquran teachers in the regions

Source: Ministry of Finance (2020).

anything, always wearing a mask, and maintaining distance) and reminding them of the discipline of carrying out health protocols.

Fourth, Rumah Zakat is a philanthropic institution that manages zakat infaq/ alms through community empowerment programmes. The empowerment programme was implemented through four prominent concepts: a champion smile (education), healthy smile (health), independent smile (economic empowerment), and sustainable smile (environmental sustainability initiative). During the COVID-19 era, the issue of food security became critical and vulnerable to Mustahiq. Therefore, in handling the COVID-19 pandemic, Rumah Zakat distributed aid through the innovative Super Qurban program (Syatar et al., 2020).

According to Senjiati and Wahyudin (2020), the SuperqUrban program produces sacrificial animals that are sold through Rumah Zakat. The innovative Rumah Zakat program was initiated in 2000 in the form of a canned sacrificial meat program with the advantage of extended durability. Senjiati and Wahyudin (2020) explained that the innovation of Rumah Zakat is in great demand by Mudhohi. The SuperqUrban program provides longer benefits, distribution to all corners of the country, affordable prices, product innovation in corned beef and canned rendang, simple processes, and voucher offers. Each corned beef box contained 40 canned beef containers with a net weight of 200 g (Senjiati & Wahyudin, 2020).

Senjiati and Wahyudin (2020) explained that the objectives of the SuperqUr-ban program are a) to reduce nutritional problems and hunger and b) Increase the fulfilment of community needs in disadvantaged, food-prone, and disaster ar-eas, especially for food procurement needs. According to Rumah Zakat (2020), SuperqUrban is distributed in villages vulnerable to nutrition and food in the re-mote areas of Indonesia and abroad. Rumah Zakat provides sustainable energy to Indonesia and the rest of the world through SuperqUrban. In addition, it supports the government in fulfilling the Sustainable Development Goals (SDGs) to end hunger, achieve food security, and improve nutrition.

With the superiority of the SuperqUrban program, aid distribution can be con-ducted throughout the year. Therefore, it can help provide nutritious food for people affected by COVID-19. For example, based on the SuperqUrban Program Report, in the January–December 2020 period, Rumah Zakat (2020) distributed 364,842 SuperqUrban cans to affected communities throughout Indonesia.

Fifth, the Paguyuban Saknah Berkah Mandiri was initiated in 2017. During the five years of the operation, the Paguyuban members reached 1,005 women. Paguy-uban's main program was to create loans using a revolving system. From the initial Indonesian Rupiah (IDR) of seven million funds, loans reached an IDR of five bil-lion. Meanwhile, the number of revolving active loans reached IDR 1.6 billion with a 100% return rate (Berkah, 2021).

This association provides economic resilience to the underprivileged families in the Antapani-Arcamanik area of Bandung. The program developed by Paguyunan SBM aimed to increase the economic resilience of low-income families. This was accomplished through a revolving funding programme. This programme uses the principles of cooperation and shared responsibility among the members of each group. During the COVID-19 era, revolving loans continued. The Paguyunan also helped work together to ease the burden on its members.

10.4   Conclusion

The COVID-19 pandemic first occurred in Wuhan, China. The WHO stated that on 26 March Indonesia's government had reported 893 cases. Poverty is one of the most influential elements of a community. It is classified as a Mustahiq. Islamic social finance exists as a solution through the collection and distribution of zakat, infaq/alms, waqf, and humanitarian aid. This study conducted inter-views, observations, and searches via the internet and reference journals to obtain data and information on the contribution of Islamic social finance in helping Mustahiq.

The study results regarding Islamic social finance found five Islamic social finance entities representing thousands of entities in Indonesia. The five entities are the National Board of Zakat (Baznas), Indonesian Waqf Board (BWI), LAZ Dewan Dakwah, LAZ Rumah Zakat, and Paguyuban Sakinah Berkah Mandiri. The results show that Islamic social finance in Indonesia contributed to the handling of

COVID-19 consequences, especially in helping Mustahiq in the form of medical equipment, food, and economic resilience.

Social finance Islamists in Indonesia have contributed to handling COVID-19. The types of funds collected by Islamic social finance include zakat funds, infaq/ alms, waqf and humanitarian donations. The funds collected are channelled to Mustahiq in various fields, including health, economy, humanity, education, and religion. Therefore, it is essential to conduct further research to examine the effects of various Islamic social finance programmes on people handling COVID-19.

The success of Islamic social finance in response to COVID-19 cannot be separated from management's various innovations. Therefore, the process of identification and exploration through further research needs to be conducted on innovation models developed by Islamic social finance in Indonesia. It is essential to gain insights into the innovation models of Islamic social finance in Indonesia.

Bibliography

Abduh, M. (2019). The role of Islamic social finance in achieving SDGs number 2: End hunger, achieve food security, improve nutrition, and promote sustainable agriculture. *Al-Shajarah, 2019* (Special Issue Islamic Banking and Finance 2019), 185–206.

Ahmed, H. (2007). Waqf -based microfinance: Realising the social role of Islamic finance "Integrating Awqaf in the Islamic financial sector." *Integrating Awqaf in the Islamic Financial Sector, 1*, 1–22.

Ainol-Basirah, A. W., & Siti-Nabiha, A. K. (2020). The roles of Islamic social finance in the era of post-COVID-19: Possible prospects of waqf Institutions for economic revival. *International Journal of Industrial Management, 7*(1), 1–8. https://doi.org/10.15282/ ijim.7.0.2020.3747

Alam, M. T. (2020). Role of Islamic finance during COVID-19: A study on practical implication of zakat as short-term emergency support system. *European Journal of Islamic Finance, 16*, 1–6. https://doi.org/10.13135/2421-2172/4581

Ascarya, A. (2020a, April). The role of integrated Islamic commercial and social finance in times of COVID-19 outbreak. *Presented in Webinar PUSKAS BAZNAS* (pp. 1–90). https://doi.org/10.13140/RG.2.2.24378.62400

Ascarya, A. (2020b). The role of Islamic social finance in times of covid-19 outbreak. *PEBS-UI, 6*, 29–30.

Azman, S. M. M. S., & Ali, E. R. A. E. (2019). Islamic social finance and the imperative for social impact measurement. *Al-Shajarah, 53*(9), 1689–1699.

Badan Amil Zakat Nasional (BAZNAS). (2019). *National Zakat Statistics.* Badan Amil Zakat Nasional. https://www.baznas.go.id

Badan Pusat Statistik. (2020). *Hasil Survei Sosial Demografi Dampak COVID-19 2020.*

Berkah, P. S. (2021). *Social Talk Paguyuban Sakinah Berlah.*

BPS Indonesia. (2020). Profil Kemiskinan di Indonesia September 2020. In *Profil Kemiskinan di Indonesia Maret, 07*(56).

Darmawan, A., & Desiana, R. (2021). Zakat dan Pemerataan Ekonomi Di Masa Pandemi COVID-19. *Al - Azhar Journal of Islamic Economics, 3*, 12–24. DOI: 10.37146/ajie. v3i1.57

Faturohman, T., Rasyid, M. F. A., Rahadi, R. A., Darmansyah, A., & Afgani, K. F. (2021). The potential role of Islamic social finance in the time of COVID-19 pandemic. *Review of Integrative Business and Economics Research, 10*(1), 95–105. http://buscompress. com/uploads/3/4/9/8/34980536/riber_10-s1_10_u20-063_95-105.pdf

Fernandes, N. (2020). Economic effects of coronavirus outbreak (COVID-19) on the world economy. *SSRN Electronic Journal*, 0–29.

Fitriani, A. (2020). The effectiveness of cash for work in handling the impact of COVID-19. *International Conference of Zakat*, 127–138. https://doi.org/10.37706/iconz.2020.235

Hafizah, G. D. (2020). Peran Ekonomi dan Keuangan Syariah pada Masa Pendemi COVID-19. *Likuid Jurnal Ekonomi Industri Halal, 1*(1-3).

Haleem, A., Javaid, M., & Vaishya, R. (2020). Effects of COVID-19 pandemic in daily life. *Current Medicine Research and Practice, 10*(2), 78–79. https://doi.org/10.1016/j.cmrp.2020.03.011

Hidayatullah, S. (2016). Wakaf Uang Dalam Perspektif Hukum Islam Dan Hukum Positif Di Indonesia. *MISYKAT: Jurnal Ilmu-Ilmu Al-Quran, Hadist, Syari'ah Dan Tarbiyah, 1*(2), 71. https://doi.org/10.33511/misykat.v1n2.71

Julia, T., Noor, A. M., & Kassim, S. (2020). Islamic social finance and green finance to achieve SDGs through minimizing post harvesting losses in Bangladesh. *Journal of Islamic Finance, 9*(2), 119–128.

Ministry of Finance. (2020). Cash waqf linked sukuk (CWLS) Seri SWR001. In *Kementrian Agama RI*, 1–14. https://bimasislam.kemenag.go.id/materiliterasi/webinar/matericwls_03.pdf

Nurjannah, & Abdulllah, M. W. (2020). Cash waqf: Economic solution during the COVID-19 pandemic. *Fitrah: Jurnal Kajian Ilmu-Ilmu Kesilaman, 6*(2), 223–242. https://doi.org/10.24952/fitrah.v6i2.3058

Obaidullah, M., & Shirazi, N. S. (2015, October). *Islamic social finance report 2015*. Islamic Research and Training Institute (IRTI).

Obaidullah, M., & Shirazi, N. S. (2017). *IRTI Islamic social finance report 2017 (1438h)*. Islamic Research and Training Institute (IRTI), 2017. https://www.researchgate.net/publication/325698377

Olanrewaju, A. S., Shahbudin, A. S. M., & Zakariyah, H. (2020). A synthesis of the Islamic social finance for sustainable Islamic social Enterprise: A four factor of production frame. *Journal of Critical Reviews, 7*(19), 9963–9974. DOI: 10.31838/jcr.07.19.1104

Pitchay, A. A., Thaker, M. A. M. T., Mydin, A. A., Azhar, Z., & Latiff, A. R. A. (2018). Cooperative-waqf model: A proposal to develop idle waqf lands in Malaysia. *ISRA International Journal of Islamic Finance, 10*(2), 225–236. https://doi.org/10.1108/IJIF-07-2017-0012

Qardawi, Y. (1973). Fiqh al Zakah. In *Mu'assat al Risalah Publishers. 2nd printing Beirut (in Arabic).*

Rizal, F., & Mukaromah, H. (2020). Filantropi Islam Solusi Atas Masalah Kemiskinan Akibat Pandemi COVID-19. *AL-MANHAJ: Jurnal Hukum Dan Pranata Sosial Islam, 3*(1), 35–66. https://doi.org/10.37680/almanhaj.v3i1.631

Sariyati, B. (2020). *Analisis distribusi zakat, infak dan sedekah dalam penanggulangan pandemi covid-19 perspektif maqashid syariah (Studi kasus BAZNAS Republik Indonesia).*

Senjiati, I. H., & Wahyudin, Y. (2020). Mudhohi's decision to implement Qurban in zakat institutions : A case study in Rumah zakat institution. *Indonesian Journal of Islamic Economics Research, 2*(2), 104–116. https://doi.org/10.18326/ijier.v2i2.4237

Susilawati, S., Falefi, R., & Purwoko, A. (2020). Impact of COVID-19's pandemic on the economy of Indonesia. *Budapest International Research and Critics Institute (BIRCI-Journal): Humanities and Social Sciences, 3*(2), 1147–1156. https://doi.org/10.33258/birci.v3i2.954

Syatar, A., Ilham, A. R. M., Mundzir, C., Arif, M., & Amiruddin, M. M. (2020). Qurban innovation due to the COVID-19: Experiences from Indonesia. *European Journal of Molecular & Clinical Medicine, 07*(10), 1600–1614.

Tahiri Jouti, A. (2019). An integrated approach for building sustainable Islamic social finance ecosystems. *ISRA International Journal of Islamic Finance, 11*(2), 246–266. https://doi.org/10.1108/IJIF-10-2018-0118

Thaker, M. A. M. T., Amin, M. F., Thaker, H. M. T., Khaliq, A., & Pitchay, A. A. (2020). Cash waqf model for micro enterprises' human capital development. *ISRA International Journal of Islamic Finance*, ahead-of-p(ahead-of-print). https://doi.org/10.1108/ ijif-08-2018-0091

WHO. (2020a). *Coronavirus disease 2019 (COVID-19) World Health Situation Report – 1*. WHO Indonesia Situation Report, 2019, 1–6.

WHO. (2020b). *Coronavirus disease 2019 (COVID-19): Situation report, 32*, 16.

Yi, B., Fen, G., Cao, D., Cai, Y., Qian, L., Li, W., Wen, Z., & Sun, X. (2021). Epidemiological and clinical characteristics of 214 families with COVID-19 in Wuhan, China. *International Journal of Infectious Diseases*. https://doi.org/10.1016/j.ijid.2021.02.021

Yumarni, A., & Suhartini, E. (2019). Optimising the role and function of Nazhir as the embodiment of accountability principle of waqf regulation in Indonesia. *Journal of Islamic Studies and Culture*, 7(2), 4–11. https://doi.org/10.15640/jisc.v7n2a2

Zain, N. R. M., & Ali, E. R. A. E. (2017). An analysis on Islamic social finance for protection and preservation of Maqāṣid Al-Sharī'ah. *Journal of Islamic Finance*, 6(Special), 133–141. https://doi.org/10.12816/0047345

Zakat, R. (2020). *Laporan Penyaluran Superqurban Periode Penyaluran Januari - Desember 2020*.

INDEX

Note:– Page references in *Italics* denotes figures and **bold** denotes tables.